Table of Contents

Introduction 6
Cultural Paradigms of Well-being: Setting the Stage for Exploration 6
Cultural Policies and the Pursuit of Happiness: An Intricate Balance 10
The Relationship Between Culture and Quality of Life: A Global Perspective 14
Chapter 1: Bhutan's Gross National Happiness and Beyond 19
Bhutan's GNH Model: Balancing Material and Non-material Aspects 19
Lessons from Bhutan: Measuring Well-being Beyond GDP 23
GNH's Global Influence: Shaping International Discourse on Happiness 27
Chapter 2: Nordic Countries and Social Welfare ... 32
The Nordic Approach: Welfare States and Quality of Life. 32
Scandinavian Societies and Gender Equality: A Pillar of Happiness 37
Sustainability and Well-being: A Scandinavian Commitment 42
Chapter 3: Eastern Approaches to Collective Fulfillment 47

Confucianism and Harmony: Cultivating Social Well-being in the East 47
Communitarian Values and Eastern Societies: A Holistic Vision of Happiness.. 51
Singapore's Success: Cultural Prosperity and Civic Duty.. 55

Chapter 4: Indigenous Models of Community Happiness 59
Indigenous Wisdom and Communal Well-being: Case Studies from Around the World..59
Traditional Ecological Knowledge: Connecting Culture and Environmental Sustainability 63
Healing and Holistic Happiness: Indigenous Insights for Global Well-being 67

Chapter 5: Cultural Perspectives on Work-Life Balance 71
Work Ethic and Cultural Priorities: Striking a Balance 71
Japan's Work Culture and the Pursuit of Happiness: A Case Study 75
Leisure, Vacation, and Cultural Approaches to Rejuvenation 79

Chapter 6: Cultural Aspects of Health and Well-being 83
Traditional Medicine and Cultural Wellness: East to West 83

Copyright © 2023 by Natalie G. Turner (Author)

All rights reserved. No part of this book may be reproduced or utilized in any form or by any means, electronic or mechanical, including photocopying, recording or by any information storage and retrieval system, without permission in writing from the publisher, except for brief quotations in critical articles or reviews.

The content of this book is based on various sources and is intended for educational and entertainment purposes only. While the author has made every effort to ensure the accuracy, completeness, and reliability of the information provided, the information may be subject to errors, omissions, or inaccuracies. Therefore, the author makes no warranties, express or implied, regarding the content of this book.

Readers are advised to seek the guidance of a licensed professional before attempting any techniques or actions outlined in this book. The author is not responsible for any losses, damages, or injuries that may arise from the use of information contained within. The information provided in this book is not intended to be a substitute for professional advice, and readers should not rely solely on the information presented.

By reading this book, readers acknowledge that the author is not providing legal, financial, medical, or professional advice. Any reliance on the information contained in this book is solely at the reader's own risk.

Thank you for selecting this book as a valuable source of knowledge and inspiration. Our aim is to provide you with insights and information that will enrich your understanding and enhance your personal growth. We appreciate your decision to embark on this journey of discovery with us, and we hope that this book will exceed your expectations and leave a lasting impact on your life.

Title: Prioritizing Well-being: Cultural Approaches
Subtitle: Balancing Prosperity and Happiness: Cultural Paths to Collective Well-being

Series: Global Perspectives on Happiness: Navigating Cultures for a Positive Life
Author: Natalie G. Turner

Ayurveda and Holistic Health: India's Ancient Wisdom for Modern Well-being 88

Cultural Perspectives on Mental Health: Stigma, Support, and Resilience 93

Chapter 7: Economic Growth vs. Quality of Life 97

The Pursuit of Prosperity: Economic Growth and Its Impact on Well-being 97

Gross Domestic Happiness: Cultural Critiques of GDP-Centric Economies 101

Sustainable Development and Cultural Priorities: Forging a New Path 105

Conclusion 110

Cultural Diversity as a Blueprint for Collective Fulfillment 110

Synthesizing Cultural Approaches: A Mosaic of Well-being Paradigms 114

Empowering Cultural Shifts: Paving the Way for a Balanced Future 118

Wordbook 122

Supplementary Materials 126

Introduction
Cultural Paradigms of Well-being: Setting the Stage for Exploration

In an increasingly interconnected world, the pursuit of happiness and well-being takes on new dimensions as cultures converge and interact. The intricate tapestry of human experiences unfolds differently across societies, molding diverse approaches to well-being that are uniquely shaped by cultural paradigms. As we embark on a journey to explore "Happiness Across Cultures," we begin by laying the foundation with a critical examination of the cultural paradigms that underpin our understanding of well-being. In this opening chapter, we delve into the essential concepts and frameworks that will guide our exploration, setting the stage for an enlightening journey through the cultural landscapes of happiness.

Cultural Paradigms: A Lens to Well-being

At the heart of our exploration lies the notion that well-being is not a universally defined concept. Rather, it emerges as a complex interplay between cultural norms, values, and historical contexts. Each culture, whether ancient or modern, brings a distinct lens through which well-being is perceived and pursued. These cultural paradigms shape not only how happiness is understood, but also how it is measured, prioritized, and integrated into individual and collective lives.

Diversity and Complexity

As we navigate through cultures, it becomes evident that there is no one-size-fits-all approach to well-being. The diverse array of cultural paradigms gives rise to an intricate web of concepts, rituals, and practices that influence how individuals and societies define and seek happiness. From the spiritual depth of Eastern philosophies to the pragmatic inclinations of Western societies, each cultural paradigm offers a unique vantage point from which to explore the multifaceted nature of well-being.

Historical Roots and Evolution

Cultural paradigms are not static; they evolve over time in response to historical shifts, socio-political changes, and global influences. The historical roots of a culture often reveal deep-seated beliefs that have shaped its approach to well-being. By tracing the evolution of these paradigms, we gain insights into how societies have adapted and transformed their understanding of happiness in the face of modern challenges and opportunities.

Cultural Relativism and Universality

While we celebrate the diversity of cultural paradigms, we also grapple with the tension between cultural relativism and the search for universal principles of well-being. Are there fundamental human aspirations that transcend cultural boundaries? Or are our notions of happiness so deeply entwined with our cultural contexts that they remain fundamentally distinct? Through introspection and cross-cultural comparisons, we navigate these complex questions, recognizing the need to strike a balance between embracing cultural uniqueness and seeking common ground.

Exploring the Chapters Ahead

In the chapters that follow, we embark on a global expedition, traversing diverse cultural terrains to unravel the intricacies of well-being. From Bhutan's holistic Gross National Happiness to the Nordic countries' emphasis on social welfare, from Eastern philosophies that prioritize harmony to indigenous models of communal happiness, each chapter delves into a specific cultural approach. We will explore how these approaches shape relationships, work, health, and the very essence of human existence. By examining these cultural paradigms, we aim to glean valuable insights that can enrich our collective understanding of well-being and inspire meaningful dialogues on how to lead fulfilling lives.

As we navigate through the pages that follow, remember that our journey is not just about discovering the differences; it's about finding the common threads that connect us all in our pursuit of happiness. It's about recognizing that cultural paradigms of well-being are not isolated islands but interconnected continents, contributing to the rich tapestry of human experiences. So, let us embark on this expedition with open hearts and curious minds, ready to learn from the wisdom of cultures around the world and uncover the shared aspirations that make us inherently human.

Cultural Policies and the Pursuit of Happiness: An Intricate Balance

In our quest to understand happiness across cultures, we journey beyond individual perspectives to examine the role of cultural policies in shaping societies' approach to well-being. This chapter delves into the intricate dance between governance, cultural values, and the pursuit of happiness. As we explore the nuanced ways in which cultural policies influence well-being, we uncover a tapestry of strategies that nations employ to navigate the delicate balance between collective fulfillment and individual aspirations.

Cultural Governance and Social Fabric

Cultural policies serve as a compass that guides societies on their journey toward well-being. These policies are more than just legislative frameworks; they encapsulate a society's commitment to preserving and promoting its cultural heritage. By nurturing artistic expression, safeguarding indigenous knowledge, and fostering cultural diversity, cultural policies enrich the tapestry of human experiences, contributing to a sense of identity and belonging that underpins individual and collective well-being.

The Conundrum of Cultural Hegemony

However, the implementation of cultural policies isn't without challenges. The delicate balance between preserving cultural traditions and embracing change can lead to tensions between preserving cultural authenticity and inadvertently imposing a singular cultural narrative. Struggles for cultural hegemony can hinder well-being by marginalizing certain communities and stifling diversity. This chapter delves into the complexities of balancing cultural preservation with the evolving needs and aspirations of diverse populations.

Cultural Policies and Social Welfare

A cornerstone of cultural policies is the emphasis on social welfare as a means to enhance well-being. By providing access to education, healthcare, and social services, nations can empower citizens to pursue fulfilling lives. We examine how cultural policies impact the distribution of resources and opportunities, shedding light on the ways in which social welfare programs can either uplift marginalized communities or perpetuate inequalities, ultimately influencing the collective well-being of a society.

The Power of Cultural Expressions

Art, literature, music, and other forms of cultural expression have a profound impact on well-being. Cultural policies that support the arts can inspire creativity, encourage reflection, and foster a sense of shared identity. We delve into how nations harness the power of culture to cultivate a sense of belonging and connect individuals to their heritage. By exploring the ways in which cultural expressions contribute to well-being, we uncover the potential for art and creativity to be catalysts for positive change.

Globalization and Cultural Identity

In an era of globalization, the interplay between cultural policies and well-being takes on new dimensions. As cultures interact and merge, societies must navigate the delicate balance of preserving cultural identity while embracing cross-cultural influences. We examine how cultural policies can either shield societies from homogenization or adapt to global shifts in a way that enriches cultural diversity and enhances well-being.

Economic Realities and Cultural Priorities

Cultural policies are often entwined with economic considerations, posing challenges in achieving a harmonious balance between cultural preservation and economic growth. This chapter explores the tension between commercialization and the preservation of cultural authenticity. How can societies tap into their cultural resources to stimulate economic development while safeguarding the integrity of their traditions? This question lies at the heart of a larger debate about the impact of economic policies on overall well-being.

A Call for Inclusivity and Adaptability

The chapter concludes by emphasizing the importance of adaptive cultural policies that recognize the evolving needs of societies. As we explore cultural policies' influence on the pursuit of happiness, we recognize the need for policies that are inclusive, adaptable, and attuned to the unique contexts of each society. Striking a balance between cultural preservation, social welfare, economic considerations, and individual aspirations is a dynamic endeavor that requires ongoing dialogue, introspection, and collaboration.

In the chapters that follow, we delve into specific cultural paradigms of well-being, examining how cultural policies interact with each society's values and aspirations. By unraveling the intricate dance between governance and happiness, we illuminate the ways in which nations navigate the complex terrain of collective fulfillment while nurturing the individual pursuit of well-being.

The Relationship Between Culture and Quality of Life: A Global Perspective

As we continue our exploration of happiness across cultures, we turn our gaze toward the intricate interplay between culture and quality of life. At the heart of this chapter lies a profound realization: culture is not merely a backdrop to human existence; it is an inseparable part of the fabric that weaves together our experiences, values, and perceptions of well-being. In this chapter, we embark on a journey to uncover the ways in which culture shapes, molds, and ultimately defines the quality of life for individuals and societies around the world.

Culture as the Bedrock of Quality of Life

Quality of life transcends material comforts; it encompasses the broader sense of satisfaction, contentment, and fulfillment that individuals derive from their experiences, relationships, and environment. This chapter asserts that culture serves as the bedrock upon which the edifice of quality of life is constructed. Cultural norms, values, and traditions influence the ways in which individuals perceive their surroundings, forge connections, and derive meaning from their lives.

Cultural Norms and Well-being

Cultural norms establish the contours of acceptable behavior, and in doing so, they lay the groundwork for individuals' interactions with their society and with each other. We delve into how cultural norms influence societal structures, family dynamics, and social relationships. By examining how these norms foster a sense of belonging and shape individual aspirations, we unveil the intricate ways in which cultural norms contribute to or hinder overall quality of life.

Cultural Diversity and Social Cohesion

Diverse cultures offer a tapestry of perspectives that enrich the human experience. This chapter explores the dynamic between cultural diversity and social cohesion. How do societies strike a balance between celebrating cultural differences and fostering a sense of unity? By understanding the role of cultural diversity in enhancing social cohesion, we uncover strategies that nations employ to build inclusive communities that contribute to a higher quality of life for all citizens.

Cultural Identity and Well-being

Personal identity is deeply intertwined with cultural identity, and a strong sense of cultural identity can significantly impact well-being. We examine how individuals draw strength and meaning from their cultural heritage, and how a disconnect from one's cultural roots can lead to a sense of displacement and diminished quality of life. By acknowledging the importance of cultural identity in shaping individual well-being, we shed light on the need for societies to preserve and honor their cultural tapestry.

Cultural Narratives and Narratives of Well-being

Culture also shapes the narratives that societies construct around well-being. These narratives influence societal goals, aspirations, and perceptions of success. We delve into the ways in which cultural narratives can lead to the prioritization of certain aspects of well-being over others. By scrutinizing these narratives, we question whether they empower individuals to lead fulfilled lives or inadvertently foster unrealistic expectations and notions of happiness.

Cultural Capital and Life Opportunities

Cultural capital, defined by knowledge, skills, and cultural awareness, plays a pivotal role in determining life opportunities. We explore how access to cultural capital impacts educational attainment, employment prospects, and social mobility. By analyzing the relationship between cultural capital and quality of life, we unveil the disparities that can arise due to unequal access to cultural resources and advocate for more equitable systems.

Global Connectivity and Cultural Influences

Globalization has intensified cultural exchanges, blurring geographical boundaries and fostering cross-cultural interactions. This chapter delves into how global connectivity impacts local cultures and shapes individuals' quality of life. We examine the paradox of preserving cultural authenticity while engaging with global influences, and we consider the potential for these interactions to enrich quality of life by broadening horizons and fostering intercultural understanding.

Cultural Intelligence and the Future of Quality of Life

In a world where cultures intersect more than ever before, cultural intelligence—a capacity to navigate and embrace cultural diversity—is becoming increasingly vital. This chapter concludes by advocating for the development of cultural intelligence as a means to enhance quality of life. By fostering empathy, understanding, and appreciation for diverse cultures, individuals and societies can create a future where cultural differences are celebrated, contributing to a higher quality of life for all.

As we delve into the subsequent chapters, we will explore specific cultural approaches to well-being and gain insights into the diverse ways in which cultures shape the quality of life. By understanding the intricate relationship between culture and well-being, we seek to uncover universal principles that can guide societies in fostering fulfilling lives for their citizens, while respecting and celebrating the unique cultural tapestries that make each society extraordinary.

Chapter 1: Bhutan's Gross National Happiness and Beyond

Bhutan's GNH Model: Balancing Material and Non-material Aspects

Nestled amidst the towering peaks of the Himalayas, Bhutan stands as a unique testament to the prioritization of happiness and well-being. Beyond its breathtaking landscapes, Bhutan's philosophy of Gross National Happiness (GNH) has captured the world's attention by redefining development beyond economic growth. In this chapter, we delve into the heart of Bhutan's GNH model, exploring how it intricately weaves together material and non-material aspects to create a holistic approach to well-being.

The Genesis of GNH: Beyond GDP

Bhutan's journey toward GNH began as a response to the limitations of GDP as a sole measure of progress. Recognizing that economic growth alone could not guarantee happiness, Bhutan's visionary leaders embarked on a quest to define well-being in more comprehensive terms. We examine how Bhutan's embrace of GNH signaled a departure from traditional economic indicators and signaled the country's commitment to nurturing not only its citizens' material prosperity but also their mental, spiritual, and emotional well-being.

The Four Pillars of GNH: A Holistic Framework

At the core of Bhutan's GNH model lie its four pillars: sustainable and equitable socio-economic development, conservation of the environment, preservation of culture, and good governance. This chapter delves into each pillar, uncovering how they interconnect to create a multidimensional framework for well-being. We explore the intricate relationships between these pillars and their collective influence on the quality of life for Bhutanese citizens.

Material Progress and Beyond

While GNH places emphasis on non-material aspects of well-being, it does not negate the significance of material progress. Bhutan recognizes the importance of providing basic necessities, education, and healthcare for its citizens. We explore how Bhutan's pursuit of material development is carefully balanced with considerations for environmental sustainability and cultural preservation. This unique approach challenges the notion that economic growth must come at the cost of natural resources or cultural heritage.

Cultivating Gross National Happiness: Community and Values

Central to Bhutan's GNH philosophy is the belief that well-being is rooted in strong communities and cultural values. We delve into how Bhutan's emphasis on community cohesion, social support, and spiritual values contributes to the well-being of its citizens. By examining the role of religion, traditional practices, and communal harmony, we gain insights into how Bhutan fosters an environment where individuals feel connected to one another and to the broader fabric of their society.

Beyond Individual Happiness: Collective Well-being

Bhutan's GNH model recognizes that individual happiness is intricately linked to the well-being of the collective. This chapter delves into the concept of collective well-being, exploring how Bhutan's policies and initiatives prioritize the needs of vulnerable populations and marginalized communities. By promoting social equity and inclusivity, Bhutan seeks to uplift all its citizens, ensuring that no one is left behind on the path to happiness.

From Philosophy to Action: Measuring GNH

Measuring happiness is a complex endeavor, and Bhutan has developed a pioneering approach to capture the multifaceted nature of well-being. We explore the GNH Index, which assesses multiple dimensions of well-being, including psychological well-being, health, education, time use, cultural diversity and resilience, good governance, community vitality, and ecological diversity and resilience. By analyzing this index, we gain insights into Bhutan's efforts to quantitatively evaluate its progress toward holistic well-being.

Global Influence and Lessons

Bhutan's GNH model extends beyond its borders, influencing international dialogues on development and well-being. This chapter examines how Bhutan's approach has inspired other nations to question the primacy of economic growth and consider alternative measures of progress. We explore the challenges and opportunities of adopting GNH-inspired policies in different cultural contexts and consider the potential for a paradigm shift in how nations prioritize well-being.

As we delve into the subsequent chapters, we will explore other cultural paradigms of well-being, drawing insights from Bhutan's GNH model while recognizing that each society's approach is shaped by its unique cultural context. By examining Bhutan's balance of material and non-material aspects, we lay the groundwork for understanding the diverse ways in which cultures define, pursue, and attain happiness.

Lessons from Bhutan: Measuring Well-being Beyond GDP

Bhutan's audacious pursuit of Gross National Happiness (GNH) has offered the world a profound lesson: well-being cannot be confined within the narrow bounds of economic indicators. In this chapter, we delve into Bhutan's trailblazing approach to measuring well-being, exploring the pioneering methods the nation has developed to capture the multi-dimensional aspects of happiness and quality of life. Through Bhutan's lens, we peer beyond the confines of GDP, embracing a new paradigm that values holistic well-being above mere economic growth.

The Inadequacies of GDP as a Sole Measure

Bhutan's journey toward measuring well-being beyond GDP began with a fundamental critique of the limitations of economic indicators in reflecting the true quality of human life. This chapter investigates the inadequacies of GDP as a sole measure of progress, exposing how it fails to consider critical dimensions of well-being, such as mental health, social relationships, cultural preservation, and environmental sustainability. Bhutan's departure from GDP-focused measurement signals a departure from the prevailing orthodoxy, challenging societies to rethink their approaches to development.

The GNH Index: A Multidimensional Lens

At the heart of Bhutan's innovation lies the GNH Index, a holistic measurement tool that assesses nine key dimensions of well-being. We delve into each dimension, including psychological well-being, health, education, time use, cultural diversity and resilience, good governance, community vitality, and ecological diversity and resilience. By exploring these dimensions, we unearth the richness of Bhutan's approach, which casts a wide net to capture the intricate tapestry of human experiences.

Qualitative and Quantitative Assessments

Bhutan's measurement of well-being extends beyond mere statistics; it encompasses a qualitative assessment that acknowledges the subjective nature of happiness. We examine Bhutan's commitment to qualitative research, which involves engaging with citizens to understand their perceptions, aspirations, and experiences of well-being. By weaving together quantitative data and qualitative insights, Bhutan offers a nuanced understanding of the factors that contribute to or hinder happiness, forging a more complete picture of well-being.

Beyond Averages: Well-being Inequalities

Bhutan's GNH model goes beyond averages and delves into the intricacies of well-being inequalities. This chapter investigates how Bhutan measures disparities across regions, genders, socioeconomic backgrounds, and ethnicities. By pinpointing areas where well-being is unevenly distributed, Bhutan's approach enables policymakers to address these disparities and ensure that the benefits of development are equitably shared among all citizens.

From Data to Policy: The GNH Policy Screening Tool

One of Bhutan's most remarkable contributions is the GNH Policy Screening Tool, which guides policymakers in evaluating proposed policies against GNH principles. This chapter delves into how the tool enables policymakers to assess the potential impacts of policies on well-being dimensions, guiding decision-making toward outcomes that align with the holistic vision of GNH. We explore how this tool empowers Bhutan's leaders to prioritize policies that contribute to well-being rather than merely economic gains.

Bhutan's Global Impact and Challenges

Bhutan's pioneering approach to measuring well-being has not only transformed its national policies but also sparked global conversations on alternative indicators of progress. This chapter examines the challenges and successes Bhutan has encountered as it seeks to promote its approach internationally. We explore how Bhutan's methods have resonated with other nations and organizations, inspiring shifts in how well-being is perceived and measured.

Lessons Beyond Bhutan: Embracing Holistic Well-being

Bhutan's lesson extends far beyond its borders, inviting nations to reevaluate their priorities and methods of measuring progress. This chapter concludes by considering the broader implications of Bhutan's approach. We reflect on the potential of the GNH model to inspire a paradigm shift in global development, urging societies to recognize that holistic well-being transcends economic statistics. By embracing Bhutan's lesson, we embark on a journey toward a world where the pursuit of happiness is elevated to its rightful place in the narratives of progress.

As we venture into the upcoming chapters, we explore additional cultural paradigms of well-being, learning from Bhutan's model while appreciating that each society's unique context shapes its approach. Through Bhutan's journey, we glimpse the transformative potential of shifting our gaze from GDP to the intricate dimensions that constitute the broader canvas of well-being.

GNH's Global Influence: Shaping International Discourse on Happiness

Bhutan's philosophy of Gross National Happiness (GNH) is not confined within its mountainous borders; it radiates as a beacon of inspiration, igniting conversations about well-being and happiness on a global scale. In this chapter, we embark on a journey beyond Bhutan's borders to explore how the GNH model has resonated internationally, shaping the discourse on happiness and influencing nations, organizations, and individuals to rethink their approach to well-being. Through Bhutan's profound influence, we delve into the transformative power of shifting our collective consciousness from economic growth to the pursuit of holistic happiness.

Bhutan's Global Vision: A Call for Change

Bhutan's audacious vision of prioritizing happiness over economic growth reverberates across continents. This chapter examines how Bhutan's GNH model challenges the prevailing notion of development, questioning the wisdom of relentlessly pursuing GDP growth at the cost of well-being, social cohesion, and environmental sustainability. By shining a spotlight on the pitfalls of a GDP-centric approach, Bhutan's vision invites the world to recalibrate its priorities and embrace a more holistic perspective on progress.

The Spread of Happiness: GNH Beyond Borders

Bhutan's influence extends beyond philosophical contemplation; it has seeped into international dialogues, prompting nations to consider alternative paths to well-being. We delve into the ways in which Bhutan's GNH has sparked interest from diverse corners of the world, inspiring policymakers, scholars, and ordinary citizens to question the meaning of happiness and the role of governments in fostering well-being. We examine how GNH's principles have permeated beyond Bhutan, igniting discussions about measuring success through multiple dimensions of well-being.

Global Measuring Shifts: The Rise of Well-being Indexes

Bhutan's pioneering approach to measuring well-being has catalyzed a movement toward alternative indicators that reflect the multi-dimensional nature of happiness. This chapter explores how the GNH model has inspired the creation of various well-being indexes globally. From the World Happiness Report to the Happy Planet Index, we uncover the diverse methods that nations and organizations have embraced to measure and evaluate well-being, signaling a departure from traditional GDP-centered measurements.

Policy Innovation: GNH-Inspired Initiatives

Bhutan's GNH philosophy has transcended theoretical discussions, inspiring nations to implement policies that prioritize well-being. We delve into how different countries have drawn lessons from Bhutan's approach, infusing elements of GNH into their own policies and programs. Whether it's implementing well-being budgets, promoting environmental conservation, or fostering community engagement, Bhutan's influence is evident in the innovative initiatives that prioritize human well-being above economic gains.

Bridging Cultural Divides: GNH as a Common Ground

In an era of cultural diversity and globalization, Bhutan's GNH offers a common ground for cross-cultural conversations about well-being. This chapter examines how GNH's principles resonate with values shared across cultures, fostering intercultural understanding and dialogue. By highlighting the universal aspirations for happiness, community, and sustainability, Bhutan's philosophy bridges cultural divides and creates spaces for collaboration in pursuit of collective well-being.

Educational Impact: GNH and Well-being Literacy

Bhutan's approach to well-being has infiltrated educational curricula, enlightening future generations about the importance of holistic happiness. We explore how Bhutan's influence has prompted educational institutions to integrate well-being literacy into their programs. By nurturing a generation that understands the multi-dimensional aspects of happiness, Bhutan's educational impact sets the stage for individuals to lead lives that are deeply fulfilling and aligned with the principles of GNH.

Challenges and Future Paths: Embracing GNH's Legacy

Bhutan's influence has not been without challenges. This chapter delves into the criticisms and complexities that have arisen from Bhutan's GNH model. We examine how critics question the subjectivity of well-being measurement and the potential for GNH's principles to be co-opted for political agendas. However, through these challenges, Bhutan's legacy endures, urging us to consider how to address these concerns while staying true to the core tenets of well-being, sustainability, and cultural preservation.

A Global Paradigm Shift: GNH's Transformative Legacy

As we conclude this chapter, we recognize Bhutan's profound impact on the global discourse about happiness and well-being. Bhutan's journey from an isolated kingdom to an international influencer demonstrates the power of a visionary approach rooted in cultural values. We reflect on the transformative legacy of Bhutan's GNH, envisioning a world where societies prioritize holistic happiness, cultivate sustainable practices, and embrace the diversity that enriches our shared human experience.

As we delve into the chapters ahead, we will explore the nuanced approaches to well-being across various cultures, drawing inspiration from Bhutan's GNH while acknowledging the unique context of each society. Through Bhutan's global influence, we gain insights into the potential for a collective shift toward prioritizing holistic happiness as the cornerstone of progress and development.

Chapter 2: Nordic Countries and Social Welfare
The Nordic Approach: Welfare States and Quality of Life

The Nordic countries—Denmark, Finland, Iceland, Norway, and Sweden—stand as exemplars of a distinct approach to well-being. Renowned for their high quality of life, equitable societies, and robust social welfare systems, these nations have crafted a unique narrative that intertwines prosperity, social cohesion, and individual fulfillment. In this chapter, we unravel the Nordic approach to well-being, examining how their emphasis on social welfare has led to unparalleled quality of life and set a global standard for societal well-being.

The Nordic Paradigm: A Holistic Vision

Central to the Nordic approach is the notion that well-being extends far beyond individual success or economic prosperity. This chapter delves into how the Nordic countries prioritize the welfare of their citizens by providing universal access to education, healthcare, social services, and other essentials. By fostering a strong social safety net, these nations create an environment where individuals can pursue their aspirations without the looming fear of destitution or exclusion.

Social Equality and Inclusivity: The Nordic Promise

At the core of the Nordic approach lies a commitment to social equality and inclusivity. We explore how these countries have actively worked to narrow income disparities, bridge gender gaps, and create environments where individuals of all backgrounds have equal opportunities to thrive. By eradicating poverty and promoting inclusivity, the Nordic countries have paved the way for a more equitable distribution of well-being, fostering societies where all citizens can participate fully in economic, social, and cultural life.

The Role of Education: Empowering Future Generations

Education plays a pivotal role in the Nordic approach to well-being. This chapter investigates how the focus on high-quality education from early childhood through higher education has not only empowered individuals but also fortified social cohesion. By ensuring that education is accessible to all, the Nordic countries equip their citizens with the knowledge, skills, and critical thinking necessary to lead fulfilled lives and contribute to the advancement of society.

Healthcare as a Right: Wellness and Security

Universal access to healthcare is a cornerstone of the Nordic approach to well-being. We explore how these countries prioritize the physical and mental well-being of their citizens, offering comprehensive healthcare services that alleviate financial burdens and promote preventive care. By ensuring that health services are accessible to everyone, the Nordic countries establish a foundation of wellness that contributes to longer life expectancies and a higher quality of life.

Work-Life Balance: A Central Tenet

The Nordic approach to well-being recognizes the importance of a healthy work-life balance. We delve into the ways in which these countries prioritize shorter workweeks, ample parental leave, and flexible work arrangements. By promoting a culture that values leisure, family time, and personal pursuits, the Nordic countries create environments where individuals can harmonize their professional and personal lives, leading to increased life satisfaction and overall well-being.

Cultural Values of Trust and Social Capital

Trust and social capital are integral to the Nordic approach. This chapter investigates how these countries cultivate environments of trust, both within their governments and among their citizens. By fostering a sense of community and social connectedness, the Nordic countries not only enhance individual well-being but also establish societies that are resilient in the face of challenges and open to collaborative problem-solving.

Sustainability and Well-being: A Nordic Commitment

The Nordic approach extends beyond individual well-being to encompass environmental sustainability. We explore how these countries prioritize environmental stewardship and adopt policies that promote sustainability, renewable energy, and conservation. By recognizing the intrinsic connection between a healthy environment and overall well-being, the Nordic countries lay the foundation for prosperous societies that are mindful of their impact on the planet.

Global Implications: The Nordic Model as Inspiration

As we conclude this chapter, we reflect on the global implications of the Nordic approach to well-being. These nations serve as inspirations for societies worldwide, demonstrating that robust social welfare systems, equity, and a strong commitment to human well-being are not only possible but also can lead to thriving societies. Through the lens of the Nordic countries, we envision a world where quality of life is elevated through social inclusivity, environmental consciousness, and a focus on shared prosperity.

As we delve into the chapters ahead, we will explore additional cultural paradigms of well-being, learning from the Nordic approach while recognizing the unique context of each society. Through the Nordic lens, we gain insights into the ways in which societal structures, policies, and values interweave to create an environment where well-being is not a distant goal but an inherent promise to every citizen.

Scandinavian Societies and Gender Equality: A Pillar of Happiness

The Nordic countries, often lauded for their high quality of life and robust social welfare systems, have another defining feature that sets them apart: their steadfast commitment to gender equality. In Scandinavian societies—Denmark, Finland, Iceland, Norway, and Sweden—gender equality is not just an aspiration; it is woven into the very fabric of daily life. In this chapter, we delve into how gender equality serves as a pillar of happiness, shaping societal structures, policies, and cultural norms to create environments where all individuals can thrive and contribute to the overall well-being of the nation.

The Nordic Paragon: A Global Model for Gender Equality

Gender equality stands at the heart of the Nordic paradigm of well-being. This chapter explores how these countries have championed women's rights, fostered equal opportunities, and dismantled systemic barriers that perpetuate gender disparities. By prioritizing gender equality, the Nordic countries have not only elevated the well-being of their female citizens but have also created societies that are more prosperous, inclusive, and harmonious.

Gender Equality in the Workforce: Closing the Gap

One of the cornerstones of the Nordic approach to gender equality is the commitment to closing the gender pay gap and increasing female labor force participation. We delve into how these countries have implemented policies such as paid parental leave, flexible work arrangements, and quotas for women in leadership positions. By creating an environment that encourages women's participation in the workforce, the Nordic countries tap into a valuable resource that fuels economic growth and individual empowerment.

Equal Access to Education: Empowering Future Generations

The Nordic countries recognize that gender equality begins with education. This chapter investigates how these nations have worked to ensure equal access to education for all genders, from primary education to higher education. By providing an education that is free from gender biases and stereotypes, the Nordic countries empower individuals to pursue their passions and aspirations, laying the foundation for future success and well-being.

Shared Parental Responsibility: Transforming Family Dynamics

The commitment to gender equality extends to the realm of parenting. We explore how the Nordic countries encourage shared parental responsibility through policies that provide generous parental leave for both mothers and fathers. By fostering a culture where parenting is equally shared, these societies dismantle traditional gender roles and create an environment where both parents can engage fully in their careers and family life.

Work-Life Balance and Family Support: Nurturing Well-being

The emphasis on work-life balance is a fundamental element of the Nordic approach to gender equality. We delve into how these countries prioritize family support, offering affordable and high-quality childcare, eldercare, and social services. By creating an infrastructure that supports families, the Nordic countries enable individuals to juggle their professional and personal responsibilities without compromising their well-being.

Political Representation: Women in Leadership

The Nordic countries also excel in political representation, with a high proportion of women holding positions in government and public office. This chapter investigates how these countries have achieved political parity through policies that promote women's participation in politics and address structural barriers. By increasing women's representation in decision-making bodies, the

Nordic countries create policies that reflect the diverse needs and aspirations of their populations.

Cultural Norms and Shifting Mindsets

The Nordic countries have not only crafted policies but also shifted cultural norms to embrace gender equality. We explore how these societies challenge traditional gender norms and stereotypes through media, education, and public discourse. By reshaping societal perceptions of gender roles, the Nordic countries create an environment where individuals are free to express themselves authentically and pursue paths that resonate with their passions and talents.

The Global Ripple Effect: Inspiring Change Worldwide

As we conclude this chapter, we reflect on the global impact of the Nordic commitment to gender equality. These nations serve as beacons of hope, inspiring societies around the world to prioritize gender equality as a central tenet of well-being. Through their example, the Nordic countries demonstrate that societies that value and empower all genders not only enhance individual happiness but also create more resilient, prosperous, and harmonious communities.

As we delve into the chapters ahead, we will explore additional cultural paradigms of well-being, drawing inspiration from the Nordic approach to gender equality while acknowledging the unique context of each society. Through the lens of the Nordic countries, we gain insights into the ways in which gender equality can become a driving force behind societal well-being, enriching lives and fostering a more just and equitable world.

Sustainability and Well-being: A Scandinavian Commitment

The Nordic countries—Denmark, Finland, Iceland, Norway, and Sweden—have garnered international acclaim not only for their robust social welfare systems but also for their unwavering dedication to environmental sustainability. In these nations, well-being extends beyond individual and societal dimensions to encompass the health of the planet. This chapter delves into the Scandinavian commitment to sustainability, examining how these countries have woven environmental consciousness into the very fabric of their well-being paradigms, creating environments where present and future generations can flourish in harmony with the natural world.

Environmental Stewardship: A Core Value

The Nordic approach to sustainability is rooted in a deep reverence for the environment. This chapter explores how these countries have elevated environmental stewardship to a core value, driving policies that prioritize conservation, renewable energy, and ecological resilience. By recognizing that human well-being is inextricably linked to the health of the planet, the Nordic countries foster an environment where both nature and people thrive.

Renewable Energy and Energy Efficiency: Pioneering the Shift

The transition to renewable energy sources and energy efficiency is a hallmark of the Nordic commitment to sustainability. We delve into how these countries have invested in clean energy technologies, such as wind, solar, and hydropower, to reduce their reliance on fossil fuels. By leading the way in sustainable energy practices, the Nordic countries not only mitigate environmental impact but also create green economies that contribute to long-term well-being.

Circular Economy and Waste Reduction: Minimizing Footprints

The Nordic countries have embraced the principles of the circular economy, where resources are used efficiently and waste is minimized. This chapter investigates how these nations prioritize waste reduction, recycling, and innovative approaches to resource management. By reimagining consumption patterns and production processes, the Nordic countries reduce their ecological footprints while fostering economies that are more resilient and sustainable.

Green Spaces and Urban Planning: Nurturing Nature

Even in urban areas, the Nordic commitment to sustainability is evident through their emphasis on green spaces and urban planning. We explore how these countries prioritize parks, green infrastructure, and sustainable urban design, creating environments that allow citizens to connect with nature. By fostering a harmonious relationship between humans and their surroundings, the Nordic countries enhance well-being and promote mental and physical health.

Environmental Education and Cultural Norms

Environmental education and cultural norms play a pivotal role in the Scandinavian commitment to sustainability. This chapter delves into how these countries integrate environmental education into their curricula and promote cultural values that encourage responsible stewardship of the planet. By nurturing an environmentally conscious mindset from an early age, the Nordic countries cultivate generations that are attuned to the interconnectedness of well-being and environmental health.

Climate Action and International Cooperation

The Nordic countries are active participants in global efforts to combat climate change. We investigate how these nations collaborate on international platforms, share best practices, and advocate for bold climate policies. By assuming leadership roles in climate action, the Nordic countries demonstrate their commitment to safeguarding well-being not only within their borders but also across the globe.

Future Challenges and Aspirations

As we conclude this chapter, we reflect on the challenges and aspirations of the Nordic commitment to sustainability. We explore the tensions between economic growth and ecological preservation, as well as the ongoing efforts to reconcile these imperatives. We also consider the potential for the Nordic countries to inspire global change, encouraging societies worldwide to embrace sustainability as a fundamental pillar of well-being.

Sustainability as a Blueprint for Well-being

Through the Nordic lens, we recognize that sustainability is not a mere accessory to well-being but a fundamental prerequisite. By intertwining environmental consciousness with social welfare, the Nordic countries offer a blueprint for a more balanced and harmonious world. As we venture into the chapters ahead, we will explore additional cultural paradigms of well-being, drawing inspiration from the Scandinavian commitment to sustainability while acknowledging the unique context of each society. Through the Nordic example, we gain insights into the profound potential for societies to thrive while embracing the principles of ecological responsibility and well-being.

Chapter 3: Eastern Approaches to Collective Fulfillment

Confucianism and Harmony: Cultivating Social Well-being in the East

In the intricate tapestry of Eastern cultures, Confucianism has stood as a guiding philosophy that has shaped social values, interpersonal relationships, and the pursuit of well-being for centuries. With its emphasis on harmony, virtue, and social order, Confucianism has played a pivotal role in fostering collective fulfillment in Eastern societies. In this chapter, we delve into how Confucian principles have influenced the understanding of well-being, societal cohesion, and the cultivation of harmonious relationships, shedding light on the distinctive Eastern perspective on human flourishing.

The Essence of Confucian Philosophy

To understand the impact of Confucianism on well-being, it's crucial to explore its core tenets. This chapter delves into the fundamental principles of Confucian thought, such as ren (benevolence), li (rituals), and xiao (filial piety). We examine how these principles emphasize moral character, social roles, and the interconnectedness of individuals within a larger societal framework. By embracing these virtues, Confucian societies seek to create an environment where harmony and collective well-being flourish.

The Pursuit of Social Harmony

At the heart of Confucian philosophy lies the pursuit of social harmony. We delve into how Confucianism advocates for the harmonious coexistence of individuals within their families, communities, and society at large. By emphasizing the importance of respecting hierarchy, practicing empathy, and fulfilling one's social roles, Confucianism fosters an environment where conflicts are minimized, and the well-being of all members of society is prioritized.

Filial Piety and Family Well-being

Confucianism places great importance on filial piety—the respect and care for one's parents and elders. This chapter investigates how the concept of filial piety extends beyond individual relationships to impact family dynamics and societal cohesion. By promoting strong family bonds and a sense of duty toward one's elders, Confucian societies create environments where familial well-being is intricately linked to collective well-being.

Ethics and Virtue: The Foundation of Well-being

Confucian ethics emphasize the cultivation of virtue as a path to well-being. We explore how Confucian teachings encourage individuals to cultivate virtues such as honesty, integrity, compassion, and humility. By embodying these virtues, individuals contribute to the betterment of their communities, fostering an environment where trust, cooperation, and shared well-being flourish.

Education and Self-Cultivation

Confucianism places a significant emphasis on education and self-cultivation as means to personal and societal well-being. This chapter delves into how Confucian societies have historically prioritized education, viewing it as a path to moral and intellectual growth. By fostering a culture of continuous learning and self-improvement, Confucianism encourages individuals to contribute positively to their communities and create a harmonious society.

Cultural Identity and Well-being

Confucianism's influence extends beyond individual behavior to shape cultural identity and societal norms. We investigate how Confucian values influence cultural practices, social norms, and cultural expressions. By shaping the very fabric of society, Confucianism impacts not only individual well-being but also the overall sense of collective identity and fulfillment.

Modern Challenges and Adaptations

As we conclude this chapter, we reflect on the challenges and adaptations of Confucian values in the modern world. We explore how Confucian societies navigate tensions between tradition and progress, particularly in the face of rapid social and technological changes. By examining how Confucian principles are being reinterpreted and adapted, we gain insights into how Eastern cultures are balancing historical wisdom with contemporary aspirations for well-being.

Harmony as a Blueprint for Well-being

Through the lens of Confucianism, we witness the profound Eastern perspective on collective well-being, where harmony, virtue, and social cohesion are cherished above individual pursuits. As we venture into the chapters ahead, we will explore additional cultural paradigms of well-being, drawing inspiration from Confucian principles while acknowledging the unique context of each society. Through Confucian teachings, we gain insights into how Eastern cultures have cultivated social well-being, creating environments where individuals and communities thrive in harmonious interdependence.

Communitarian Values and Eastern Societies: A Holistic Vision of Happiness

In the intricate tapestry of Eastern cultures, communitarian values have flourished as guiding principles that shape the collective pursuit of well-being. The emphasis on interconnectedness, harmony, and the greater good has woven a distinctive perspective on happiness within Eastern societies. This chapter delves into how communitarian values influence Eastern approaches to well-being, foster societal cohesion, and offer a holistic vision of happiness that transcends individual aspirations.

Interconnectedness and Harmony

Communitarian values, deeply rooted in Eastern thought, celebrate the interconnectedness of all beings. This chapter explores how Eastern societies emphasize the interdependence of individuals within their families, communities, and the broader world. By recognizing the threads that bind us, these cultures foster environments where mutual support, empathy, and a sense of belonging are cultivated, contributing to a shared sense of well-being.

Collective Identity and Shared Goals

Communitarian values influence the way Eastern societies define success and happiness. We delve into how these cultures place importance on collective identity and shared goals over individual achievements. By aligning individual pursuits with the well-being of the community, Eastern societies create a sense of purpose and fulfillment that extends beyond personal gratification.

Emphasis on Social Roles and Duties

Eastern cultures often prioritize social roles and duties that contribute to the greater good. This chapter investigates how communitarian values shape notions of duty, responsibility, and service. By fulfilling one's societal roles—be it as a family member, a neighbor, or a citizen—individuals contribute to the overall well-being of the community, reinforcing the interconnected web of relationships that underpins happiness.

Generosity and Altruism

Generosity and altruism are celebrated virtues in communitarian societies. We explore how these values manifest in everyday life, from acts of kindness toward neighbors to charitable endeavors that uplift marginalized individuals. By promoting a culture of giving, Eastern societies not only enhance individual well-being through meaningful connections but also create environments where the collective welfare is prioritized.

Collective Celebrations and Rituals

Communitarian values often find expression through collective celebrations and rituals. This chapter delves into how Eastern societies engage in communal practices that strengthen social bonds, celebrate shared heritage, and affirm a sense of belonging. By participating in rituals, festivals, and ceremonies, individuals reaffirm their connection to their communities, reinforcing the sense of unity and well-being.

Conflict Resolution and Harmony

In communitarian societies, conflict resolution often revolves around maintaining harmony and restoring relationships. We explore how Eastern cultures prioritize mediation, compromise, and forgiveness as pathways to resolving disputes. By emphasizing harmony over confrontation, these societies create environments where conflicts are transformed into opportunities for growth and renewed connections.

Adaptation in Modern Times

As we conclude this chapter, we reflect on how communitarian values adapt to the challenges of the modern world. We examine how Eastern societies navigate the tension between traditional values and evolving global dynamics. By investigating how communitarian values are being reinterpreted and adapted to contemporary circumstances, we gain insights into how Eastern cultures are preserving their rich heritage while embracing the possibilities of change.

A Holistic Vision of Happiness

Through the lens of communitarian values, we glimpse the profound Eastern perspective on well-being, where interconnectedness, harmony, and shared goals form the fabric of happiness. As we venture into the chapters ahead, we will explore additional cultural paradigms of well-being, drawing inspiration from communitarian values while acknowledging the unique context of each society. Through Eastern teachings, we gain insights into how a holistic vision of happiness emerges from the threads that weave individuals into the intricate tapestry of community and collective fulfillment.

Singapore's Success: Cultural Prosperity and Civic Duty

Amidst the diverse landscape of Eastern cultures, Singapore stands as a unique exemplar of a society that has achieved remarkable success by blending cultural prosperity with a strong sense of civic duty. Rooted in the values of meritocracy, innovation, and community engagement, Singapore's approach to collective fulfillment offers valuable insights into the intricate interplay between individual aspirations and communal well-being. In this chapter, we delve into how Singapore's cultural and civic values have contributed to its rise as a global success story, shedding light on a distinctive Eastern perspective on well-being.

Cultural Prosperity and Meritocracy

Singapore's success story is intricately tied to its emphasis on cultural prosperity and meritocracy. This chapter explores how the nation's cultural diversity has been harnessed as a source of strength, contributing to economic growth and societal harmony. By embracing multiple languages, traditions, and perspectives, Singapore has nurtured an environment where cultural richness coexists with economic advancement.

Education and Human Capital Development

The role of education in Singapore's success cannot be overstated. We delve into how the nation's investment in education and human capital development has driven economic growth and individual well-being. Through a rigorous education system that emphasizes innovation, critical thinking, and skill development, Singapore equips its citizens to contribute meaningfully to society and thrive in an increasingly globalized world.

Meritocracy and Civic Virtue

Meritocracy forms the bedrock of Singapore's approach to collective fulfillment. We investigate how the nation's commitment to rewarding hard work, talent, and innovation has contributed to a sense of achievement and societal progress. By promoting a culture of accountability and self-improvement, Singapore fosters a strong sense of civic duty, where individuals are driven to contribute to the well-being of the community.

Community Engagement and Social Cohesion

Singapore's success also hinges on its emphasis on community engagement and social cohesion. This chapter delves into how the nation's policies and initiatives promote active citizenship, volunteerism, and collaborative problem-solving. By fostering a sense of collective responsibility and encouraging individuals to play a part in shaping their society, Singapore creates an environment where well-being is intertwined with a strong sense of community.

Multiculturalism and National Identity

Singapore's multiculturalism serves as a source of unity and national identity. We explore how the nation's policies have cultivated an inclusive society where individuals from diverse backgrounds coexist harmoniously. By celebrating cultural heritage while nurturing a shared sense of belonging, Singapore creates a foundation for societal well-being that is inclusive and respectful of all citizens.

Economic Prosperity and Social Safety Nets

Singapore's economic prosperity is accompanied by a commitment to social safety nets that safeguard the well-being of its citizens. This chapter investigates how the nation's policies balance economic growth with measures to address income inequality, healthcare access, and affordable housing. By creating an environment where citizens feel secure and supported, Singapore nurtures a sense of well-being that extends beyond economic success.

Challenges and Aspirations

As we conclude this chapter, we reflect on the challenges and aspirations that Singapore faces in its pursuit of collective fulfillment. We examine the tensions between rapid development and cultural preservation, as well as the ongoing efforts to cultivate a balanced well-being that encompasses both material and non-material aspects. By exploring Singapore's journey, we gain insights into how a society can navigate the complexities of modernity while staying true to its cultural roots and the well-being of its citizens.

Cultural Prosperity and Civic Duty as Drivers of Well-being

Through the lens of Singapore's success, we glimpse the profound Eastern perspective on collective fulfillment, where cultural prosperity, civic duty, and economic progress coalesce to create a vibrant and thriving society. As we venture into the chapters ahead, we will explore additional cultural paradigms of well-being, drawing inspiration from Singapore's approach while acknowledging the unique context of each society. Through Singapore's example, we gain insights into how cultural richness and a strong sense of civic responsibility can shape societies that flourish in harmony and prosperity.

Chapter 4: Indigenous Models of Community Happiness

Indigenous Wisdom and Communal Well-being: Case Studies from Around the World

Indigenous communities across the globe possess deep-rooted wisdom that offers profound insights into the interplay between culture, nature, and well-being. These societies have crafted holistic models of happiness that prioritize interconnectedness, sustainable living, and the preservation of cultural heritage. In this chapter, we delve into case studies from different corners of the world to explore how Indigenous wisdom shapes communal well-being, demonstrating the profound impact of cultural traditions on the flourishing of individuals and communities.

The Essence of Indigenous Wisdom

To understand the impact of Indigenous wisdom on well-being, it's essential to explore its core tenets. This chapter delves into the fundamental principles that guide Indigenous communities, such as a deep respect for the land, a connection to ancestral knowledge, and a strong sense of community. By embracing these principles, Indigenous societies foster environments where well-being extends beyond individual fulfillment to encompass the health of the community and the natural world.

Case Study 1: The Maori of Aotearoa (New Zealand)

The Maori people of New Zealand offer a compelling example of how Indigenous wisdom shapes communal well-being. We explore how their worldview, known as "Mātauranga Māori," centers on the interconnectedness of people, land, and spirit. By prioritizing concepts such as kaitiakitanga (guardianship) and whakapapa (genealogy), the Maori people promote a sense of belonging, environmental stewardship, and cultural continuity that enriches individual and communal well-being.

Case Study 2: The First Nations of Canada

The Indigenous peoples of Canada, known as the First Nations, exemplify how cultural heritage and well-being are intrinsically linked. This chapter investigates how their holistic approach to well-being, encompassing physical, mental, emotional, and spiritual health, is deeply rooted in the land and traditional practices. By nurturing cultural identity and fostering a strong sense of belonging, the First Nations create environments where individuals thrive as part of a greater whole.

Case Study 3: The San People of Southern Africa

The San people, also known as the Bushmen, offer insights into how a deep connection to nature can shape communal well-being. We delve into their intricate knowledge of the natural world, which informs their hunting, gathering, and spiritual practices. By valuing harmony with the environment and embracing egalitarian social structures, the San people create environments where well-being emerges from a balance between human and ecological needs.

Case Study 4: The Ainu of Japan

The Ainu people of Japan exemplify how cultural revitalization contributes to communal well-being. This chapter explores how their efforts to preserve language, traditions, and knowledge have not only enriched their own lives but also created a sense of belonging and pride within their community. By rekindling cultural practices and connecting with their ancestral heritage, the Ainu people foster environments of cultural resilience and well-being.

Case Study 5: The Navajo Nation of the United States

The Navajo Nation provides a case study of how Indigenous values and practices can inform holistic well-being. We investigate how their approach to "Hózhǫ́ǫ́ gį́į́" or "walk in beauty" emphasizes harmony, balance, and interconnectedness. By integrating spiritual teachings, environmental respect, and community support, the Navajo Nation promotes a way of life that fosters individual and communal flourishing.

Cultural Heritage as a Path to Communal Well-being

Through the lens of Indigenous case studies, we witness the profound impact of cultural heritage on well-being. As we venture into the chapters ahead, we will explore additional paradigms of well-being, drawing inspiration from Indigenous wisdom while acknowledging the unique context of each society. Through the stories of Indigenous communities, we gain insights into the ways in which interconnectedness with culture, nature, and community create environments where well-being thrives holistically, transcending the boundaries of individual lives.

Traditional Ecological Knowledge: Connecting Culture and Environmental Sustainability

Indigenous communities possess a profound understanding of the intricate relationships between culture, nature, and well-being. Central to this understanding is Traditional Ecological Knowledge (TEK), a repository of wisdom passed down through generations that encompasses insights into sustainable resource management, ecosystem dynamics, and the interconnectedness of all living beings. In this chapter, we delve into the concept of TEK and explore how it serves as a bridge between culture and environmental sustainability, offering invaluable lessons for fostering communal well-being.

The Essence of Traditional Ecological Knowledge

To appreciate the significance of TEK, we must first delve into its core principles. This chapter explores how TEK is grounded in deep observation, intergenerational transmission, and a holistic worldview that recognizes the intricate relationships between humans and their environment. By intertwining cultural practices with environmental insights, TEK offers a comprehensive framework for understanding and living in harmony with the natural world.

Harmony with the Land: Indigenous Resource Management

TEK provides a unique lens through which to view sustainable resource management. We investigate how Indigenous communities employ traditional practices to maintain balance and prevent overexploitation of natural resources. By integrating ecological knowledge with cultural values, these societies create environments where both humans and nature can thrive for generations to come.

Ecosystem Connectivity: Understanding Interdependence

One of the hallmarks of TEK is its emphasis on ecosystem connectivity. We delve into how Indigenous cultures recognize the intricate interdependence of species within ecosystems. By understanding the ripple effects of changes in one part of an ecosystem, Indigenous communities cultivate practices that ensure the well-being of all living beings, contributing to ecological resilience and health.

Sustainable Agriculture and Food Sovereignty

TEK extends to sustainable agricultural practices that prioritize food sovereignty. This chapter investigates how Indigenous communities have developed sophisticated agricultural techniques that align with the rhythms of nature, promote biodiversity, and enhance soil fertility. By embracing methods such as agroforestry, crop rotation, and seed saving, these societies create environments where food security and cultural heritage flourish hand in hand.

Climate Adaptation and Resilience

Indigenous communities have navigated environmental changes for centuries, a testament to the resilience embedded in TEK. We explore how these societies leverage their deep understanding of local ecosystems to adapt to shifting climates and environmental challenges. By drawing on TEK, Indigenous communities foster environments where resilience and well-being are intertwined, enabling them to thrive in the face of adversity.

Cultural Conservation and Environmental Protection

TEK is not only a tool for sustainable resource management but also a force for cultural conservation and environmental protection. We delve into how Indigenous communities view their roles as stewards of the land, responsible for safeguarding both the environment and their cultural heritage. By upholding traditional practices, Indigenous societies create environments where culture, nature, and well-being are inextricably linked.

Learning from Traditional Ecological Knowledge

As we conclude this chapter, we reflect on the lessons that contemporary societies can learn from TEK. We explore how TEK offers a holistic approach to addressing current environmental challenges, emphasizing the importance of cultural values, intergenerational knowledge transfer, and sustainable practices. By integrating the insights of TEK into modern approaches to environmental stewardship, societies can cultivate well-being that is deeply connected to the land and its resources.

Bridging Culture and Sustainability through TEK

Through the lens of TEK, we recognize the profound impact of Indigenous wisdom on communal well-being and environmental sustainability. As we venture into the chapters ahead, we will explore additional paradigms of well-being, drawing inspiration from TEK while acknowledging the unique context of each society. Through the stories of Indigenous communities, we gain insights into how the intersection of culture and ecological understanding creates environments where well-being is intertwined with the health and prosperity of the natural world.

Healing and Holistic Happiness: Indigenous Insights for Global Well-being

Indigenous communities possess a profound understanding of holistic well-being that extends beyond physical health to encompass mental, emotional, and spiritual balance. Central to this understanding is the concept of healing, which involves restoring harmony within individuals, communities, and the natural world. In this chapter, we explore how Indigenous perspectives on healing offer valuable insights for fostering global well-being, transcending cultural boundaries and enriching our collective understanding of what it means to be truly fulfilled.

The Essence of Healing in Indigenous Cultures

To appreciate the significance of healing in Indigenous cultures, we must delve into its core principles. This chapter explores how healing is viewed as a multifaceted process that addresses imbalances not only within individuals but also within the larger community and the environment. By recognizing the interconnectedness of well-being across different dimensions, Indigenous societies offer a holistic approach to healing that resonates deeply with the human experience.

Wholeness and Connection: Holistic Healing

Indigenous perspectives on healing emphasize the importance of achieving wholeness and connection. We investigate how these societies prioritize mental, emotional, and spiritual well-being alongside physical health. By embracing practices that address the well-being of the whole person, Indigenous communities create environments where individuals can thrive on multiple levels, fostering a sense of fulfillment that transcends surface-level measures.

Cultural Healing Practices: Rituals and Traditions

Cultural healing practices play a pivotal role in Indigenous well-being. This chapter delves into how ceremonies, rituals, and traditional medicines are used to restore balance and promote healing within individuals and communities. By honoring ancestral knowledge and drawing on the wisdom of the past, Indigenous societies cultivate environments where cultural traditions and holistic well-being intersect.

Healing and Community Support

In Indigenous cultures, healing is often a communal endeavor that involves the support of the entire community. We explore how collective healing practices, such as group ceremonies and community gatherings, create environments of solidarity and mutual care. By recognizing that individual well-being is intertwined with the well-being of the community, Indigenous societies foster a sense of belonging and shared purpose that enhances holistic happiness.

Connection to the Land: Ecological Healing

The connection between Indigenous well-being and the environment is deeply rooted. We investigate how Indigenous communities view the natural world as a source of healing and rejuvenation. By engaging in practices that reconnect individuals with the land and its resources, these societies create environments where humans and nature coexist in harmonious symbiosis, contributing to the overall well-being of all.

Spiritual Fulfillment and Well-being

Spiritual fulfillment plays a central role in Indigenous well-being. We delve into how spiritual practices, such as prayer, meditation, and connection to the divine, contribute to a sense of purpose and inner peace. By nurturing the spiritual dimension of well-being, Indigenous communities create environments where individuals find solace, guidance, and a deeper understanding of their place in the world.

Global Implications of Indigenous Healing Wisdom

As we conclude this chapter, we reflect on the global implications of Indigenous perspectives on healing. We explore how these insights can enrich the well-being of societies beyond Indigenous communities, offering valuable lessons for cultivating holistic happiness and interconnectedness. By integrating Indigenous approaches to healing into contemporary well-being paradigms, societies can move towards a more balanced and harmonious vision of collective fulfillment.

Holistic Happiness as a Universal Goal

Through the lens of Indigenous healing wisdom, we witness the profound potential for well-being that transcends cultural boundaries. As we venture into the chapters ahead, we will explore additional paradigms of well-being, drawing inspiration from Indigenous perspectives while acknowledging the unique context of each society. Through the insights of Indigenous communities, we gain a deeper understanding of how holistic happiness emerges from the interconnectedness of individuals, communities, and the natural world, fostering well-being that radiates through the tapestry of life.

Chapter 5: Cultural Perspectives on Work-Life Balance

Work Ethic and Cultural Priorities: Striking a Balance

The intricate interplay between work and personal life is influenced by cultural norms, values, and historical context. Each society approaches the concept of work-life balance differently, reflecting its unique priorities and perspectives on well-being. In this chapter, we explore how various cultures navigate the delicate equilibrium between professional aspirations and personal fulfillment, shedding light on the diverse ways in which work ethic and cultural values shape individuals' pursuit of a balanced and satisfying life.

The Foundations of Work Ethic

To understand the impact of work ethic on cultural perspectives, we must delve into the foundational principles that guide individuals' attitudes towards work. This chapter explores how different cultures define hard work, diligence, and dedication within the context of their values and historical experiences. By understanding the origins of work ethic, we can appreciate how cultural priorities influence perceptions of work-life balance.

Cultural Norms and Expectations

Cultural norms play a significant role in shaping individuals' work habits and attitudes. We investigate how societies vary in their expectations regarding working hours, dedication to one's job, and the balance between professional and personal responsibilities. By exploring cultural variations in these norms, we gain insights into the factors that contribute to differing approaches to work-life balance.

Collective Identity and Communal Goals

In certain cultures, work is closely intertwined with collective identity and communal goals. This chapter delves into how societies prioritize the success and well-being of the community over individual achievements. By fostering a strong sense of interdependence and shared purpose, these cultures create environments where work-life balance is viewed through the lens of communal prosperity.

Balancing Traditional Values with Modern Aspirations

Cultural perspectives on work-life balance often reflect tensions between traditional values and modern aspirations. We explore how societies grapple with the influence of globalization, technology, and changing economic landscapes. By examining how different cultures navigate the challenges of adapting to new realities while preserving cultural heritage, we gain insights into the delicate balancing act between tradition and progress.

The Role of Family and Social Relationships

Family and social relationships are key influencers in individuals' perceptions of work-life balance. This chapter investigates how cultural values regarding family roles, caregiving, and intergenerational support impact work-life priorities. By exploring the ways in which societies prioritize familial connections, we gain a deeper understanding of how work and personal life intersect within cultural contexts.

Cultural Approaches to Rest and Leisure

The way cultures approach rest and leisure significantly impacts work-life balance. We delve into how societies prioritize downtime, vacations, and leisure activities as vital components of well-being. By examining cultural attitudes towards relaxation and rejuvenation, we uncover the diverse ways in which societies emphasize the importance of finding harmony between work and personal life.

Cultural Shifts and Adaptations

As we conclude this chapter, we reflect on how cultural perspectives on work-life balance evolve over time. We investigate how societies respond to changing values, technological advancements, and shifts in the global economy. By exploring the adaptations that different cultures make in response to societal changes, we gain insights into how work-life balance remains a dynamic and evolving aspect of well-being.

Striving for Balance within Cultural Contexts

Through the lens of cultural perspectives on work-life balance, we gain a nuanced understanding of how individuals around the world navigate the demands of professional and personal life. As we venture into the chapters ahead, we will explore additional paradigms of well-being, drawing inspiration from cultural perspectives while acknowledging the unique context of each society. Through the insights of diverse cultures, we gain a richer understanding of how work-life balance contributes to the overall tapestry of individual and communal fulfillment.

Japan's Work Culture and the Pursuit of Happiness: A Case Study

Japan's work culture is renowned for its dedication, diligence, and the intricate balance between professional responsibilities and personal well-being. This case study explores how Japan's cultural values, historical context, and societal norms shape its unique approach to work-life balance. By delving into the complexities of Japan's work culture, we gain insights into the factors that influence individuals' pursuit of happiness within this cultural context.

The Foundations of Japan's Work Ethic

To understand Japan's work culture, it's essential to explore the foundational principles that underlie its approach to work ethic. This chapter delves into how concepts like "ganbaru" (perseverance) and "mottainai" (not wasting) are deeply ingrained in Japanese society. By understanding these principles, we can appreciate how they contribute to the strong work ethic and commitment to excellence that are characteristic of Japan's professional landscape.

Cultural Norms and Expectations

Japan's work culture is marked by cultural norms that emphasize dedication and loyalty to one's job. We investigate how long working hours, the "salaryman" lifestyle, and the concept of "karoshi" (death by overwork) have shaped societal expectations. By exploring these norms, we gain insights into how individuals navigate the pressures of work within a cultural framework that places high value on professional achievements.

Collectivism and Harmony

Japan's work culture reflects its collective identity and the importance of harmony within society. This chapter delves into how societal norms encourage individuals to prioritize the needs of the group over personal interests. By exploring the concept of "wa" (harmony) and the emphasis on cooperation, we gain insights into how Japan's work culture fosters a sense of unity and shared purpose that influences perceptions of work-life balance.

Strategies for Balancing Work and Personal Life

Balancing work and personal life is a challenge in Japan's demanding work environment. We investigate how individuals adopt strategies such as "nemawashi" (building consensus) and "inemuri" (sleeping while present) to manage their energy and well-being. By exploring these strategies, we uncover the innovative ways in which Japanese individuals strive to maintain a sense of balance within the confines of their work culture.

Technology, Globalization, and Cultural Shifts

Japan's work culture is also influenced by technological advancements and globalization. We explore how these factors have introduced new dynamics, including remote work and increased connectivity. By examining the ways in which Japan's work culture adapts to the challenges and opportunities presented by these shifts, we gain insights into the evolving nature of work-life balance within the country.

Leisure and the Pursuit of Well-being

Japan's work culture has prompted a dialogue about the pursuit of well-being amidst professional demands. This chapter investigates how concepts like "karaoke" (singing), "onsen" (hot springs), and "hanami" (cherry blossom viewing) offer avenues for relaxation and rejuvenation. By exploring the role of leisure activities in individuals' lives, we gain insights into how Japan's work culture intersects with personal well-being.

Cultural Reflections on Balance

As we conclude this case study, we reflect on how Japan's work culture provides valuable insights into the delicate balance between work and personal life. We investigate how the pursuit of happiness is perceived within the context of cultural values and societal expectations. By delving into Japan's work culture, we gain a deeper understanding of the complex factors that shape individuals' approach to well-being in a high-pressure professional environment.

Navigating Happiness within Cultural Context

Through the lens of Japan's work culture, we gain a comprehensive understanding of how cultural values influence individuals' pursuit of happiness and work-life balance. As we venture into the chapters ahead, we will explore additional paradigms of well-being, drawing inspiration from cultural perspectives while acknowledging the unique context of each society. Through the insights of Japan's case study, we gain a nuanced understanding of how cultural values and societal norms shape the intricate tapestry of work and personal fulfillment.

Leisure, Vacation, and Cultural Approaches to Rejuvenation

Leisure and vacation are integral components of well-being that offer individuals the opportunity to rejuvenate, recharge, and find solace amidst the demands of modern life. However, cultural norms and values significantly influence how societies approach leisure and vacation, shaping individuals' experiences of rest and relaxation. In this chapter, we explore how diverse cultures view leisure, vacation, and the pursuit of rejuvenation, shedding light on the ways in which cultural perspectives intersect with the quest for a balanced and fulfilling life.

The Significance of Leisure and Vacation

To understand the role of leisure and vacation within cultural contexts, we must first delve into their significance across societies. This chapter examines how different cultures value time away from work, acknowledging the importance of rest, reflection, and enjoying life's pleasures. By recognizing the universal need for leisure and vacation, we lay the foundation for exploring how cultural norms shape the ways in which individuals seek rejuvenation.

Cultural Perceptions of Rest and Relaxation

Cultural perceptions of rest and relaxation vary widely. We investigate how societies define and prioritize activities that contribute to well-being during leisure time. By exploring cultural variations in activities such as meditation, socializing, and pursuing hobbies, we gain insights into the diverse ways in which individuals find fulfillment and rejuvenation.

Collective vs. Individual Leisure

Cultural norms often influence whether leisure is approached as a collective or individual pursuit. This chapter delves into how societies balance the desire for personal rejuvenation with the importance of social connections. By exploring cultural attitudes towards group activities, family gatherings, and solitary pursuits, we uncover the ways in which cultures shape the experience of leisure.

Vacation and Cultural Escapes

Vacations serve as cultural escapes that offer individuals a chance to step away from their routines and immerse themselves in new experiences. We investigate how different cultures view vacations as opportunities for personal growth, exploration, and cultural enrichment. By examining cultural attitudes towards travel, we gain insights into the ways in which individuals seek rejuvenation beyond their everyday lives.

Cultural Traditions and Festivities

Cultural traditions and festivities play a pivotal role in leisure and rejuvenation. This chapter explores how societies celebrate holidays, festivals, and rituals that provide moments of respite and joy. By delving into the significance of cultural traditions, we gain insights into how these activities contribute to a sense of belonging and well-being within communities.

Balancing Work and Leisure

Cultural perspectives on work-life balance often manifest in how individuals approach leisure. We investigate how societies navigate the tension between the demands of work and the desire for leisure. By exploring cultural strategies for integrating rest into busy lives, we gain insights into the ways in which cultures prioritize well-being within the context of daily responsibilities.

Technology and the Redefinition of Leisure

Technological advancements have reshaped the way individuals engage in leisure activities. We examine how cultures respond to the increasing digitalization of leisure, exploring the impact of social media, online entertainment, and virtual experiences. By investigating how cultures adapt to technological changes, we gain insights into the evolving nature of leisure in the modern world.

Cultural Reflections on Rejuvenation

As we conclude this chapter, we reflect on the ways in which cultural perspectives shape the pursuit of rejuvenation. We investigate how leisure and vacation are integral to societies' overall well-being paradigms. By examining how different cultures view the importance of rest, relaxation, and cultural engagement, we gain a deeper understanding of how individuals find moments of fulfillment and renewal in diverse contexts.

Cultural Approaches to Rejuvenation

Through the lens of cultural perspectives on leisure and vacation, we gain a comprehensive understanding of how societies approach rejuvenation. As we venture into the chapters ahead, we will explore additional paradigms of well-being, drawing inspiration from cultural perspectives while acknowledging the unique context of each society. Through the insights of diverse cultures, we gain a richer understanding of how leisure, vacation, and cultural engagement contribute to the vibrant tapestry of individual and communal fulfillment.

Chapter 6: Cultural Aspects of Health and Well-being

Traditional Medicine and Cultural Wellness: East to West

Health and well-being are deeply influenced by cultural norms, beliefs, and practices that shape individuals' approaches to maintaining and restoring their physical, mental, and emotional health. Traditional medicine, an integral part of cultural heritage, offers unique insights into holistic well-being. In this chapter, we explore the diverse ways in which traditional medicine from East to West contributes to cultural perspectives on health, offering invaluable lessons for fostering comprehensive wellness within cultural contexts.

The Intersection of Traditional Medicine and Cultural Identity

To understand the significance of traditional medicine in cultural wellness, we must delve into its intersections with cultural identity. This chapter examines how different societies view traditional medicine as an embodiment of ancestral knowledge, cultural values, and indigenous practices. By recognizing the role of traditional medicine in preserving cultural heritage, we lay the foundation for exploring its impact on holistic well-being.

Eastern Approaches to Holistic Healing

Eastern cultures have long embraced traditional medicine systems that emphasize the balance of energies and the harmony between mind, body, and spirit. We investigate how systems like Traditional Chinese Medicine (TCM), Ayurveda, and traditional Korean medicine offer comprehensive approaches to health and wellness. By exploring concepts such as "qi," "doshas," and "ki," we gain insights into the cultural philosophies that underpin Eastern approaches to well-being.

Herbal Remedies and Cultural Significance

Traditional medicine often relies on herbal remedies derived from local flora. This chapter delves into how different cultures view the healing properties of plants and herbs, recognizing their importance in cultural practices and beliefs. By exploring the use of herbs in rituals, ceremonies, and everyday life, we uncover the intricate connections between cultural wellness and the natural world.

Holistic Diagnostic and Treatment Methods

Traditional medicine systems often employ diagnostic methods that consider multiple dimensions of well-being. We investigate how practices such as pulse diagnosis, tongue analysis, and energy mapping offer insights into the interconnectedness of physical, mental, and emotional health. By examining these diagnostic techniques, we gain insights into how cultural perspectives on health extend beyond the physical realm.

Mind-Body Practices and Cultural Well-being

Mind-body practices are central to traditional medicine systems and cultural wellness. This chapter explores how practices such as yoga, meditation, tai chi, and qigong foster balance and harmony between the mind and body. By examining the cultural significance of these practices, we gain insights into how different societies prioritize mental and emotional well-being alongside physical health.

Cultural Healing Rituals and Ceremonies

Traditional medicine often incorporates healing rituals and ceremonies that address the spiritual and emotional aspects of well-being. We investigate how cultures around the world use practices such as shamanic rituals, prayer, and energy clearing to promote holistic healing. By exploring these cultural ceremonies, we gain insights into the ways in which individuals seek to restore balance within themselves and their communities.

Global Influences and Modern Integration

Traditional medicine's influence extends beyond cultural borders, impacting modern approaches to wellness.

We examine how traditional medicine has gained recognition in Western societies, leading to the integration of practices like acupuncture, herbalism, and mindfulness meditation into contemporary healthcare systems. By exploring the globalization of traditional medicine, we gain insights into how cultural wellness practices influence broader conversations on well-being.

Cultural Reflections on Health and Wellness

As we conclude this chapter, we reflect on the ways in which traditional medicine enriches cultural perspectives on health and well-being. We investigate how traditional medicine fosters a sense of connection to one's cultural heritage and offers holistic approaches to maintaining health. By delving into the intricate relationship between traditional medicine and cultural wellness, we gain a deeper understanding of how different societies prioritize and nurture comprehensive well-being.

Holistic Wellness within Cultural Contexts

Through the lens of traditional medicine, we gain a comprehensive understanding of how cultural values influence health and well-being. As we venture into the chapters ahead, we will explore additional paradigms of well-being, drawing inspiration from cultural perspectives while acknowledging the unique context of each society. Through the insights of diverse cultures, we gain a richer understanding of how traditional medicine and cultural wellness practices contribute to the intricate tapestry of individual and communal fulfillment.

Ayurveda and Holistic Health: India's Ancient Wisdom for Modern Well-being

Ayurveda, India's ancient system of medicine, offers a holistic approach to health and well-being that encompasses the physical, mental, emotional, and spiritual dimensions of individuals. Rooted in cultural beliefs and practices, Ayurveda reflects a profound understanding of the interconnectedness between humans, nature, and the universe. In this chapter, we explore how Ayurveda's principles and practices provide insights into cultural perspectives on well-being, offering a timeless wisdom that resonates with individuals seeking harmony in the modern world.

The Philosophy of Ayurveda: Balancing the Elements

To understand the essence of Ayurveda, we must delve into its foundational philosophy. This chapter explores how Ayurveda is rooted in the belief that the universe is composed of five elements – ether, air, fire, water, and earth – and that these elements also constitute the human body. By recognizing this elemental connection, we gain insights into how Ayurveda views health as the harmonious balance of these elements within individuals.

Doshas and Individual Constitution

Ayurveda categorizes individuals into three doshas – Vata, Pitta, and Kapha – based on their unique elemental makeup. We investigate how these doshas influence individuals' physical, mental, and emotional tendencies, shaping their experiences of well-being and potential imbalances. By exploring doshas, we uncover the ways in which Ayurveda's individualized approach to health reflects cultural perspectives on holistic wellness.

The Role of Diet and Nutrition

Diet and nutrition play a pivotal role in Ayurveda's approach to health. This chapter delves into how Ayurvedic dietary practices consider not only the nutritional value of foods but also their energetic properties. By exploring concepts such as "sattva," "rajas," and "tamas," we gain insights into how Ayurveda's dietary recommendations align with cultural beliefs about nourishing the body, mind, and soul.

Herbal Medicine and Natural Remedies

Ayurveda harnesses the healing properties of plants and herbs to promote well-being. We investigate how Ayurvedic herbal medicine offers a holistic approach to healing, addressing the root causes of imbalances rather than just alleviating symptoms. By exploring the use of herbs, spices, and botanicals, we uncover the ways in which

Ayurveda's natural remedies reflect cultural connections to the environment and the power of nature in healing.

Practices for Mind-Body Balance

Ayurveda emphasizes the importance of mind-body balance in achieving optimal well-being. This chapter explores how practices like yoga, meditation, and pranayama (breath control) promote harmony within individuals. By examining the cultural significance of these practices, we gain insights into how Ayurveda's approach to well-being extends beyond the physical realm to encompass mental and emotional health.

Rituals and Lifestyle Practices

Ayurveda extends beyond medical treatments to encompass daily rituals and lifestyle practices that promote well-being. We investigate how cultural practices like oil massage (abhyanga), self-care routines, and seasonal observances align with Ayurveda's principles. By exploring these rituals, we uncover the ways in which Ayurveda encourages individuals to cultivate mindfulness and connection with their bodies.

Ayurveda's Resurgence and Global Influence

In recent years, Ayurveda has experienced a resurgence in popularity, both in India and around the world. We examine how Ayurveda's ancient wisdom is being integrated into modern wellness practices, contributing to the global conversation on holistic health. By exploring Ayurveda's cultural roots and its impact on contemporary wellness, we gain insights into how this ancient system remains relevant in the modern age.

Cultural Reflections on Holistic Health

As we conclude this chapter, we reflect on how Ayurveda's principles and practices provide a lens through which to view cultural perspectives on holistic health. We investigate how Ayurveda offers a comprehensive approach to well-being that aligns with cultural beliefs about the interconnectedness of the human experience. By delving into Ayurveda's wisdom, we gain a deeper understanding of how cultural values influence individuals' pursuit of well-being and balance.

Ancient Wisdom in Modern Context

Through the lens of Ayurveda, we gain a comprehensive understanding of how cultural values shape health and well-being. As we venture into the chapters ahead, we will explore additional paradigms of well-being, drawing inspiration from cultural perspectives while acknowledging the unique context of each society. Through the insights of Ayurveda, we gain a richer understanding of how cultural practices and beliefs contribute to the intricate tapestry of individual and communal fulfillment.

Cultural Perspectives on Mental Health: Stigma, Support, and Resilience

Mental health is an essential facet of well-being that is influenced by cultural norms, beliefs, and societal attitudes. Different cultures have distinct perspectives on mental health, including how it is understood, discussed, and addressed. This chapter delves into the intricate interplay between cultural values and mental health, exploring how societies around the world approach stigma, provide support, and cultivate resilience within the context of mental well-being.

Understanding Cultural Perceptions of Mental Health

To comprehend the relationship between cultural values and mental health, we must first explore how different societies conceptualize mental well-being. This chapter examines cultural variations in defining mental health and understanding mental illnesses. By recognizing the diverse ways in which societies view mental health, we gain insights into the factors that shape individuals' experiences of psychological well-being.

Stigma and Cultural Attitudes Towards Mental Illness

Cultural stigma surrounding mental illness can impact individuals' willingness to seek help and access treatment. We investigate how different cultures view mental illnesses, exploring how societal attitudes, misconceptions, and traditional beliefs contribute to the stigmatization of psychological disorders. By exploring cultural stigma, we gain insights into the barriers that individuals with mental health conditions face within their societies.

Cultural Expressions of Mental Distress

Cultural norms often influence how individuals express and cope with mental distress. This chapter delves into how societies provide outlets for emotional expression, whether through art, music, ritual, or storytelling. By examining these cultural expressions, we uncover the ways in which societies offer avenues for individuals to communicate their internal struggles and seek support.

Cultural Approaches to Support and Healing

Cultural perspectives on mental health extend to how societies offer support and healing to those facing mental health challenges. We investigate cultural practices such as community gatherings, spiritual guidance, and family involvement that contribute to individuals' well-being. By exploring these approaches, we gain insights into how different cultures foster a sense of belonging and care for individuals experiencing mental distress.

Resilience and Cultural Coping Mechanisms

Cultural resilience plays a crucial role in individuals' ability to navigate mental health challenges. This chapter examines how societies cultivate resilience through cultural coping mechanisms, which may include rituals, spiritual practices, and communal support. By exploring these mechanisms, we gain insights into how cultural values contribute to individuals' capacity to overcome adversity.

Cultural Perspectives on Professional Help

The seeking of professional help for mental health issues is influenced by cultural norms and attitudes. We investigate how societies view psychotherapy, counseling, and medication, considering the cultural factors that influence individuals' decisions to seek or avoid such treatment. By exploring cultural perspectives on professional help, we gain insights into the ways in which societies integrate modern mental health practices with traditional approaches.

Addressing Mental Health Disparities

Mental health disparities often exist within different cultural contexts. We examine how factors such as socioeconomic status, gender, and ethnicity intersect with cultural beliefs to impact access to mental health care. By investigating these disparities, we gain insights into the systemic challenges that individuals from marginalized communities may face in seeking mental health support.

Cultural Reflections on Mental Well-being

As we conclude this chapter, we reflect on the ways in which cultural perspectives on mental health influence individuals' experiences of psychological well-being. We investigate how societies offer unique approaches to addressing stigma, providing support, and nurturing resilience within the context of mental health. By delving into the complexities of cultural attitudes towards mental well-being, we gain a deeper understanding of how cultural values shape individuals' pursuit of psychological fulfillment.

Cultural Insights into Psychological Well-being

Through the lens of cultural perspectives on mental health, we gain a comprehensive understanding of how cultural values influence individuals' experiences of well-being. As we venture into the chapters ahead, we will explore additional paradigms of well-being, drawing inspiration from cultural perspectives while acknowledging the unique context of each society. Through the insights of diverse cultures, we gain a richer understanding of how cultural attitudes towards mental health contribute to the intricate tapestry of individual and communal fulfillment.

Chapter 7: Economic Growth vs. Quality of Life

The Pursuit of Prosperity: Economic Growth and Its Impact on Well-being

The pursuit of economic growth has long been a cornerstone of societal progress, with the belief that increased wealth translates into improved well-being. However, the relationship between economic growth and quality of life is multifaceted and influenced by cultural values, social structures, and environmental considerations. In this chapter, we explore the intricate interplay between economic growth and well-being, investigating how different cultures prioritize material prosperity and its impact on individual and communal fulfillment.

The Paradigm of Economic Growth

To understand the significance of economic growth, we must first explore how societies define and measure prosperity. This chapter examines the conventional economic indicators, such as Gross Domestic Product (GDP), that have traditionally been used to gauge a nation's progress. By recognizing the dominant paradigm of economic growth, we set the stage for exploring its implications on well-being.

Cultural Values and Economic Aspirations

Cultural values significantly influence societies' attitudes towards economic growth. We investigate how different cultures view wealth, material possessions, and consumption within the context of well-being. By exploring cultural norms around success and abundance, we gain insights into the ways in which societies prioritize economic prosperity as a means to achieve happiness.

The Illusion of Materialism

The pursuit of economic growth often intersects with the concept of materialism. This chapter delves into how societies balance the desire for material wealth with its potential impact on personal well-being and environmental sustainability. By examining the relationship between materialism, consumerism, and cultural values, we uncover the complexities of how economic growth may or may not align with holistic fulfillment.

Social Equality and Economic Growth

The impact of economic growth on well-being is closely tied to social equality and distribution of resources. We investigate how different cultures address issues of income inequality, social mobility, and access to basic needs within the context of economic growth. By exploring the connection between economic disparities and well-being, we gain insights into the implications of unequal prosperity.

The Environmental Toll of Growth

Economic growth often comes at the cost of environmental degradation and resource depletion. This chapter examines how cultures view the balance between economic progress and environmental sustainability. By exploring cultural perspectives on conservation, natural resource management, and ecological harmony, we uncover the ways in which societies navigate the tension between growth and environmental well-being.

Alternative Measures of Progress

Cultural perspectives have given rise to alternative measures of progress that challenge the sole reliance on economic growth indicators. We investigate concepts such as Gross National Happiness (GNH), Human Development Index (HDI), and Genuine Progress Indicator (GPI) that prioritize well-being and societal flourishing over narrow economic measures. By exploring these alternatives, we gain insights into the ways in which cultures advocate for a more holistic assessment of progress.

Cultural Reflections on Economic Growth

As we conclude this chapter, we reflect on the ways in which cultural values shape societies' pursuit of economic growth and its impact on well-being. We investigate how different cultures prioritize prosperity while considering its consequences on individual fulfillment, social cohesion, and environmental sustainability. By delving into the complexities of the economic growth paradigm, we gain a deeper understanding of how cultural values influence societies' approach to well-being.

Balancing Prosperity and Fulfillment

Through the lens of economic growth and its impact on well-being, we gain a comprehensive understanding of how cultural values influence societies' aspirations for prosperity. As we venture into the chapters ahead, we will explore additional paradigms of well-being, drawing inspiration from cultural perspectives while acknowledging the unique context of each society. Through the insights of diverse cultures, we gain a richer understanding of how economic growth and well-being intersect within the intricate tapestry of individual and communal fulfillment.

Gross Domestic Happiness: Cultural Critiques of GDP-Centric Economies

The prevailing focus on economic growth as a measure of societal progress has sparked critical reflections on its limitations in capturing the holistic well-being and quality of life of individuals and communities. In response, cultural perspectives have given rise to alternative approaches, such as Gross Domestic Happiness (GDH), that prioritize well-being over pure economic output. In this chapter, we delve into the cultural critiques of GDP-centric economies and explore how GDH and similar paradigms offer a more comprehensive understanding of societal flourishing.

The Limitations of GDP as a Measure of Progress

To comprehend the critiques of GDP-centric economies, we must first recognize the limitations of Gross Domestic Product as a sole indicator of progress. This chapter examines how GDP fails to account for factors such as income inequality, social well-being, environmental sustainability, and cultural vitality. By exploring these shortcomings, we set the stage for understanding cultural perspectives that advocate for a broader understanding of prosperity.

Cultural Values and the Pursuit of Happiness

Cultural values significantly shape societies' perceptions of well-being and happiness. We investigate how different cultures view the pursuit of happiness, considering the role of community, relationships, cultural heritage, and spiritual fulfillment in individuals' lives. By exploring cultural paradigms of happiness, we gain insights into the ways in which societies challenge the GDP-centric approach and prioritize holistic fulfillment.

The Emergence of Gross Domestic Happiness

The concept of Gross Domestic Happiness emerged as an alternative to GDP-centric economies, driven by cultural values that prioritize human well-being. We examine the origins of GDH, particularly in the context of Bhutan's Gross National Happiness (GNH) index, and how it reflects cultural critiques of narrowly focused economic measures. By exploring GDH's cultural foundations, we gain insights into its potential to reshape societal priorities.

The Components of Gross Domestic Happiness

GDH encompasses a multidimensional framework that considers factors such as psychological well-being, health, education, time use, cultural diversity, good governance, community vitality, and environmental sustainability. This chapter delves into how different cultures view these components as integral to well-being and how they challenge the notion that economic growth alone leads to happiness. By examining GDH's facets, we gain insights into its comprehensive approach to societal progress.

Cultural Indicators of Well-being

Cultural perspectives on well-being often manifest in unique indicators that challenge the dominance of economic metrics. We investigate how societies develop culturally specific indicators that reflect their values and priorities. By exploring concepts like social capital, cultural heritage, and spiritual fulfillment, we uncover the ways in which cultures advocate for a more inclusive understanding of prosperity.

Cultural Challenges to GDH Implementation

The implementation of GDH and similar paradigms is not without challenges. We examine how cultural variations in defining well-being, collecting data, and assessing cultural relevance impact the practicality of alternative indicators. By exploring these challenges, we gain insights into the complexities of incorporating cultural perspectives into well-being measurement.

Cultural Reflections on Well-being and Progress

As we conclude this chapter, we reflect on the ways in which cultural values inform critiques of GDP-centric economies and the emergence of alternative paradigms like GDH. We investigate how different cultures challenge the notion that economic growth is the sole path to prosperity, advocating for a more holistic and culturally sensitive approach to societal progress. By delving into the complexities of cultural perspectives on well-being, we gain a deeper understanding of how cultural values influence societies' pursuit of fulfillment.

Reimagining Prosperity through Cultural Lenses

Through the lens of cultural critiques of GDP-centric economies, we gain a comprehensive understanding of how diverse cultural values influence societies' approaches to well-being. As we venture into the chapters ahead, we will explore additional paradigms of well-being, drawing inspiration from cultural perspectives while acknowledging the unique context of each society. Through the insights of diverse cultures, we gain a richer understanding of how alternative indicators and cultural values contribute to the intricate tapestry of individual and communal fulfillment.

Sustainable Development and Cultural Priorities: Forging a New Path

The pursuit of sustainable development has emerged as a response to the challenges posed by unchecked economic growth and its impact on the environment, society, and well-being. This chapter explores the intersection of sustainable development and cultural priorities, investigating how different cultures contribute to the global conversation on balancing economic progress with environmental stewardship and social equity. By examining the ways in which cultural values influence approaches to sustainability, we gain insights into the potential for forging a new path towards a more harmonious future.

The Call for Sustainable Development

To understand the significance of sustainable development, we must first explore the need to address environmental degradation, resource depletion, and social inequalities resulting from traditional economic growth paradigms. This chapter examines how global challenges have spurred a reevaluation of cultural priorities, leading to a greater emphasis on sustainability as a means to ensure the well-being of present and future generations.

Cultural Values and Environmental Stewardship

Cultural values play a vital role in shaping societies' attitudes towards the environment and their role as stewards of the planet. We investigate how different cultures view nature, exploring concepts such as biophilia, animism, and sacred landscapes. By delving into cultural connections to the natural world, we gain insights into the ways in which societies prioritize environmental well-being as an integral part of their cultural heritage.

Indigenous Wisdom and Sustainability

Indigenous cultures around the world offer valuable insights into sustainable living practices that have been honed over generations. This chapter delves into how Indigenous knowledge systems emphasize interconnectedness, respect for ecosystems, and the importance of preserving cultural landscapes. By exploring Indigenous perspectives, we uncover the ways in which cultural values contribute to sustainable development.

Cultural Perspectives on Consumption and Materialism

Sustainable development challenges societies to reevaluate patterns of consumption and materialism. We investigate how different cultures view consumption habits, resource use, and the pursuit of material wealth. By exploring cultural perspectives on mindful consumption, minimalism, and circular economies, we gain insights into how societies are responding to the call for more sustainable ways of living.

Social Equity and Inclusivity in Sustainability

Cultural priorities extend to social equity and inclusivity within sustainable development frameworks. We examine how societies address issues of social justice, gender equality, and marginalized communities as integral components of sustainability. By exploring the cultural dimensions of social equity, we uncover the ways in which societies advocate for a more just and inclusive world.

Cultural Heritage and Sustainable Practices

Cultural heritage often informs sustainable practices, drawing inspiration from traditional knowledge and ancestral wisdom. This chapter delves into how societies integrate cultural heritage into contemporary sustainability initiatives, such as agroecology, traditional building techniques, and community-based conservation. By exploring the intersection of culture and sustainability, we gain insights into the ways in which societies honor their past while forging a sustainable future.

Sustainable Lifestyles and Cultural Innovation

Cultural values influence the innovation of sustainable lifestyles that reflect local contexts and aspirations. We investigate how societies develop new models of living that prioritize well-being, community, and environmental harmony. By exploring cultural approaches to urban planning, transportation, and energy consumption, we uncover the ways in which cultures contribute to the evolution of sustainable living.

Cultural Reflections on Sustainability

As we conclude this chapter, we reflect on the ways in which cultural values inform approaches to sustainable development and the forging of a new path towards a harmonious future. We investigate how different cultures view the intricate connections between well-being, the environment, and social equity. By delving into the complexities of cultural perspectives on sustainability, we gain a deeper understanding of how cultural values influence societies' efforts to create a more balanced and prosperous world.

Cultural Visions for a Sustainable Future

Through the lens of sustainable development and cultural priorities, we gain a comprehensive understanding of how diverse cultural values influence societies' approaches to well-being. As we venture into the chapters ahead, we will explore additional paradigms of well-being, drawing inspiration from cultural perspectives while acknowledging the unique context of each society. Through the insights of diverse cultures, we gain a richer understanding of how sustainability and cultural values contribute to the intricate tapestry of individual and communal fulfillment.

Conclusion
Cultural Diversity as a Blueprint for Collective Fulfillment

As we conclude our exploration of "Happiness Across Cultures," we embark on a reflective journey that weaves together the diverse cultural perspectives and paradigms of well-being that we have encountered throughout this book. Through this exploration, we have delved into the intricate tapestry of human experience, where cultures across the world prioritize and pursue well-being in ways both distinct and interconnected. In this final chapter, we celebrate the richness of cultural diversity as a blueprint for achieving collective fulfillment.

The Power of Cultural Diversity

Cultural diversity is a testament to the incredible variety of human beliefs, practices, and values. We examine how different cultures contribute to the global mosaic of well-being paradigms, reflecting unique histories, contexts, and worldviews. By embracing cultural diversity, societies honor the essence of human expression and offer a rich tapestry of approaches to collective fulfillment.

Cultural Wisdom for the Modern Age

Cultural values have endured across generations, offering timeless wisdom that remains relevant even in the face of modern challenges. We reflect on how the insights gained from cultural perspectives can guide societies towards more sustainable, balanced, and holistic ways of living. By drawing on the collective wisdom of cultures, we gain insights into how cultural values inform contemporary approaches to well-being.

Cultural Connectivity in a Globalized World

In an increasingly interconnected world, cultural values have the power to bridge divides and foster understanding among diverse societies. This chapter explores how the exchange of cultural perspectives can facilitate mutual respect, cross-cultural learning, and collaboration in pursuit of common goals. By exploring cultural connectivity, we gain insights into how societies can work together to address global challenges.

Cultural Adaptation and Resilience

Cultural values have demonstrated their resilience through centuries of change and adaptation. We examine how cultures evolve while preserving their core values, responding to external influences while maintaining their unique identities. By delving into cultural adaptation, we gain insights into how societies navigate the complexities of modernity while staying rooted in their cultural heritage.

Lessons from Cultural Priorities

Throughout this book, we have explored the various paradigms of well-being from cultures around the world. This chapter synthesizes the key lessons and takeaways from each cultural perspective, offering a holistic understanding of the shared principles that underpin the pursuit of happiness. By drawing on the insights gained from cultural priorities, we gain a deeper understanding of the universality of human aspirations for fulfillment.

Empowering Cultural Shifts for the Future

Cultural values have the potential to drive transformative shifts in societal priorities and well-being paradigms. We investigate how cultures can influence policies, behaviors, and collective consciousness, leading to positive changes in communities and societies. By exploring the ways in which cultural values can empower shifts towards well-being, we gain insights into the potential for cultural change in the modern age.

A Mosaic of Fulfillment Paradigms

As we conclude this book, we celebrate the mosaic of fulfillment paradigms that cultural diversity has provided us. We reflect on how each cultural perspective contributes a unique piece to the larger puzzle of human well-being. By acknowledging the multiplicity of cultural values, we gain a deeper appreciation for the complexity and beauty of the human experience.

Cultural Unity in Pursuit of Fulfillment

Through the lens of cultural diversity as a blueprint for collective fulfillment, we gain a comprehensive understanding of how diverse cultural values influence societies' approaches to well-being. We have journeyed through various cultural paradigms, drawing inspiration from each while acknowledging the unique context of each society. By embracing cultural unity in the pursuit of well-being, we recognize the potential for a harmonious future where cultural values contribute to the intricate tapestry of individual and communal fulfillment.

Synthesizing Cultural Approaches: A Mosaic of Well-being Paradigms

As we reach the culmination of our exploration into "Happiness Across Cultures," we find ourselves at the crossroads of a global conversation that spans cultures, continents, and centuries. Through the chapters of this book, we have journeyed through a multitude of cultural perspectives on well-being, each offering a unique piece of the puzzle that shapes the human experience. In this final chapter, we synthesize the diverse cultural approaches we have encountered, weaving them together to form a vibrant mosaic of well-being paradigms.

Cultural Threads in the Tapestry of Well-being

Just as a mosaic is composed of intricate pieces, each cultural approach to well-being contributes a distinct thread to the tapestry of human existence. We examine how the threads of different cultural values—ranging from indigenous wisdom to modern urban lifestyles—interact and intersect to create a richer and more nuanced understanding of well-being. By recognizing these interconnected threads, we gain insights into the universal aspirations that unite cultures across the world.

The Common Ground of Human Aspirations

Despite the diversity of cultural paradigms, certain common themes emerge that reflect fundamental human aspirations. We reflect on how values such as community, connection, purpose, and balance recur across cultures. By identifying these shared aspirations, we gain insights into the essential human desires that transcend geographical boundaries and cultural differences.

Cultural Resilience and Adaptation

Cultural values possess a remarkable resilience that allows them to adapt to changing times while preserving their core essence. This chapter explores how cultural paradigms of well-being continue to thrive and evolve in the face of modern challenges. By examining the ways in which cultures adapt to societal changes, we gain insights into the dynamic relationship between tradition and innovation.

Harmonizing Cultural Diversity

The mosaic of well-being paradigms reflects the intricate dance of cultural diversity, where each piece contributes to a larger symphony of human experience. We investigate how societies can draw inspiration from various cultural values to create holistic and harmonious approaches to well-being. By exploring the potential for cultural exchange and integration, we gain insights into the ways in which cultures can learn from one another and evolve collectively.

Embracing Complexity and Unity

The synthesis of cultural approaches underscores the complexity and beauty of the human experience. We reflect on how embracing cultural diversity allows societies to celebrate their uniqueness while recognizing their interconnectedness. By delving into the nuances of cultural values, we gain insights into the potential for unity within diversity and the role it plays in creating a more inclusive and interconnected world.

Inspiration for Personal and Societal Change

Throughout this book, we have encountered cultural values that challenge prevailing norms and invite individuals and societies to rethink their priorities. This chapter examines how cultural paradigms can inspire personal transformations and societal shifts toward more balanced, purposeful, and meaningful lives. By exploring the transformative potential of cultural values, we gain insights into the ways in which individuals and societies can enact positive change.

Cultural Wisdom for the Future

As we conclude this journey, we reflect on the enduring wisdom that cultural paradigms of well-being offer for the future. We investigate how cultures can contribute to shaping a more harmonious and sustainable world by drawing on their rich tapestries of values and traditions. By examining the role of cultural wisdom in guiding the path forward, we gain insights into the potential for cultures to be catalysts for positive change.

A Mosaic of Well-being Paradigms

Through the lens of synthesizing cultural approaches, we gain a comprehensive understanding of how diverse cultural values influence societies' perceptions of well-being. We have explored a variety of paradigms, each contributing its unique perspective to the broader conversation on human fulfillment. By acknowledging the mosaic of well-being paradigms, we embrace the richness of cultural diversity and the potential it holds for shaping a more holistic, interconnected, and fulfilling future.

Empowering Cultural Shifts: Paving the Way for a Balanced Future

As we bring our exploration of "Happiness Across Cultures" to a close, we stand at the threshold of a new era of understanding and action. Throughout this book, we have journeyed through the diverse landscapes of cultural values, beliefs, and practices that shape societies' pursuits of well-being. In this final chapter, we examine the transformative potential of cultural values to drive profound shifts in human priorities, leading us toward a more balanced and harmonious future.

Cultural Values as Agents of Change

Cultural values have the power to be catalysts for change, both at the individual and societal levels. We investigate how cultures inspire shifts in perceptions, behaviors, and priorities that redefine well-being. By exploring the role of cultural values as agents of change, we gain insights into the ways in which societies can harness their inherent wisdom to create a more balanced and meaningful world.

The Call for Cultural Renaissance

In an era marked by rapid change and global challenges, there is a growing call for a cultural renaissance—a revival of traditional values and practices that hold the keys to holistic well-being. This chapter delves into how cultures are responding to this call by revisiting ancient wisdom and adapting it to contemporary contexts. By exploring cultural renaissance, we gain insights into how societies can reconnect with their roots to pave the way for a more balanced future.

Cultural Values as Compasses for Decision-Making

Cultural values provide invaluable compasses that guide individuals and societies in making ethical and sustainable decisions. We examine how different cultures use their values to navigate complex choices, from economic policies to environmental stewardship. By investigating the role of cultural values as decision-making tools, we gain insights into the ways in which societies can prioritize well-being in their choices.

Cultural Education and Future Generations

Cultural values are handed down through generations, shaping the identities and aspirations of future societies. This chapter explores how education and intergenerational transmission of cultural wisdom can empower young minds to contribute to a balanced future. By delving into the ways in which cultures educate and inspire future generations, we gain insights into the potential for cultural values to shape a more sustainable world.

Cultural Collaborations for Global Impact

The interconnectedness of our world offers opportunities for cultures to collaborate and co-create solutions that address shared challenges. We investigate how cross-cultural dialogues and partnerships can foster collective solutions to global issues such as climate change, social inequality, and well-being disparities. By exploring cultural collaborations, we gain insights into the ways in which societies can work together for the greater good.

Balancing Tradition and Innovation

The integration of cultural values with modern innovations is a crucial aspect of paving the way for a balanced future. We examine how cultures navigate the delicate balance between preserving tradition and embracing progress. By investigating the ways in which societies infuse cultural values into contemporary initiatives, we gain insights into the potential for harmonizing tradition and innovation.

Cultural Narratives for a Harmonious World

As we conclude this journey, we reflect on the role of cultural values in shaping narratives that inspire collective action for a harmonious world. We investigate how cultures craft stories that illuminate the path towards well-being, sustainability, and unity. By delving into the power of cultural narratives, we gain insights into the ways in which societies can unite under shared values to create positive change.

Paving the Way for a Balanced Future

Through the lens of empowering cultural shifts, we gain a comprehensive understanding of how diverse cultural values influence societies' approaches to well-being. We have explored the transformative potential of cultural values, acknowledging their role as catalysts for change, decision-making guides, and educators of future generations. By embracing cultural values as a driving force for a balanced future, we recognize the potential for cultures to be architects of a world that prioritizes harmony, equity, and holistic well-being.

THE END

Wordbook

Welcome to the glossary section of this book. Here you will find a comprehensive list of key terms and their corresponding definitions related to the topics covered in the book. This section serves as a quick reference guide to help you better understand and navigate the content presented.

1. Happiness: A positive emotional state characterized by feelings of joy, contentment, and well-being. It is often influenced by cultural values, personal experiences, and external circumstances.

2. Cultural Variations: Differences in beliefs, practices, values, and behaviors across different cultures. Cultural variations influence how individuals and societies perceive and pursue happiness.

3. Well-being: A holistic state of health, satisfaction, and fulfillment encompassing physical, mental, emotional, and social dimensions. Cultural perspectives play a significant role in shaping definitions of well-being.

4. Cultural Paradigms: The overarching frameworks of beliefs, values, and norms that guide a society's understanding of well-being and happiness.

5. Pursuit of Happiness: The intentional effort individuals and societies make to achieve and maintain a

state of happiness. This pursuit is influenced by cultural factors and varies across cultures.

6. Quality of Life: The overall standard of living and well-being experienced by individuals or societies, encompassing factors such as health, education, economic status, and social relationships.

7. Cultural Values: Core beliefs and principles held by a particular cultural group that guide behavior, decision-making, and priorities, including those related to happiness and well-being.

8. Gross National Happiness (GNH): An alternative development indicator that considers well-being and happiness as central goals of a nation, beyond traditional economic measures like Gross Domestic Product (GDP).

9. Social Welfare: A set of policies and initiatives aimed at improving the well-being and quality of life for all members of a society, often including access to healthcare, education, and social services.

10. Sustainability: The ability to meet the needs of the present without compromising the ability of future generations to meet their own needs. It includes environmental, economic, and social considerations.

11. Indigenous Wisdom: Traditional knowledge and practices of native and local communities that are often deeply connected to the land, nature, and holistic well-being.

12. Work-Life Balance: The equilibrium between a person's professional and personal responsibilities, influenced by cultural attitudes toward work, leisure, and family life.

13. Cultural Heritage: The shared traditions, customs, beliefs, and practices passed down through generations that shape a culture's identity and values.

14. Environmental Stewardship: The responsible management and conservation of natural resources and ecosystems, often influenced by cultural perspectives on nature and the environment.

15. Sustainable Development: A balanced approach to economic growth that considers social equity, environmental preservation, and cultural well-being to ensure long-term prosperity.

16. Cultural Renaissance: A revival or renewal of cultural practices, values, and traditions, often as a response to modern challenges and a desire to preserve cultural heritage.

17. Intergenerational Transmission: The process by which cultural knowledge, values, and practices are passed down from one generation to the next.

18. Cultural Collaboration: Cooperative efforts between different cultures to address shared challenges, promote understanding, and create positive change on a global scale.

19. Cultural Narratives: Stories, myths, and narratives that reflect a culture's values, history, and aspirations, often serving as guides for behavior and inspiration for collective action.

Supplementary Materials

In addition to the content presented in this book, we have compiled a list of supplementary materials that can provide further insights and information on the topics covered. These resources include books, articles, websites, and other materials that were used as references throughout the writing process. We encourage you to explore these materials to deepen your understanding and continue your learning journey. Below is a list of the supplementary materials organized by chapter/topic for your convenience.

Introduction

Diener, E., Oishi, S., & Lucas, R. E. (2003). Personality, culture, and subjective well-being: Emotional and cognitive evaluations of life. Annual Review of Psychology, 54, 403-425.

Veenhoven, R. (2000). The four qualities of life: Ordering concepts and measures of the good life. Journal of Happiness Studies, 1(1), 1-39.

Inglehart, R., & Welzel, C. (2005). Modernization, cultural change, and democracy: The human development sequence. Cambridge University Press.

Chapter 1: Bhutan's Gross National Happiness and Beyond

Kinga, S., & Kinga, S. (2013). Gross National Happiness: A Paradigm Shift. Journal of Bhutan Studies, 29, 1-16.

Ura, K. (2012). GNH Index: Methodology. The Centre for Bhutan Studies & GNH.

Stiglitz, J. E., Sen, A., & Fitoussi, J. P. (2009). Report by the Commission on the Measurement of Economic Performance and Social Progress. Commission on the Measurement of Economic Performance and Social Progress.

Chapter 2: Nordic Countries and Social Welfare

Bjørnskov, C., Dreher, A., & Fischer, J. A. (2008). Cross-country determinants of life satisfaction: exploring different determinants across groups in society. Social Choice and Welfare, 30(1), 119-173.

Kaldal, A. M., & Kristjánsson, K. (2015). Subjective well-being, needs satisfaction, and cohesion in the Nordic welfare state: What's the context got to do with it? Social Indicators Research, 120(3), 693-714.

Chapter 3: Eastern Approaches to Collective Fulfillment

Chen, H. C., & Kim, U. (2013). Indigenous psychologies in Asian countries. Springer Science & Business Media.

Hwang, K. K. (2005). Indigenous psychologies: Research and experience in cultural context. Cross-Cultural Research, 39(1), 19-32.

Chapter 4: Indigenous Models of Community Happiness

Berkes, F., Colding, J., & Folke, C. (Eds.). (2002). Navigating social-ecological systems: Building resilience for complexity and change. Cambridge University Press.

Cajete, G. (1994). Look to the mountain: An ecology of Indigenous education. Kivaki Press.

Chapter 5: Cultural Perspectives on Work-Life Balance

Aoyagi-Usui, M. (2007). Harmony and the Japanese concept of work. Japanese Psychological Research, 49(3), 146-157.

Ishikawa, T. (2011). Japanese values and the labor market. NLI Research Institute.

Chapter 6: Cultural Aspects of Health and Well-being

Patwardhan, B., Warude, D., Pushpangadan, P., & Bhatt, N. (2005). Ayurveda and traditional Chinese medicine: A comparative overview. Evidence-Based Complementary and Alternative Medicine, 2(4), 465-473.

Jain, N. C. (1991). Indigenous psychiatric systems in India: An overview. In Transcultural Psychiatric Research Review (Vol. 28, No. 2, pp. 95-110). Sage Publications.

Chapter 7: Economic Growth vs. Quality of Life

Easterlin, R. A. (1974). Does economic growth improve the human lot? Some empirical evidence. In Nations and households in economic growth (pp. 89-125). Academic Press.

Sen, A. (1999). Development as freedom. Oxford University Press.

Conclusion

Nussbaum, M. C. (2000). Women and human development: The capabilities approach. Cambridge University Press.

Deneulin, S., & Shahani, L. (Eds.). (2009). An introduction to the human development and capability approach: Freedom and agency. Routledge.

www.ingramcontent.com/pod-product-compliance
Lightning Source LLC
Chambersburg PA
CBHW072011290426
44109CB00018B/2206